Riding the Infertility Roller Coaster

by

Iris Waichler, MSW, LCSW

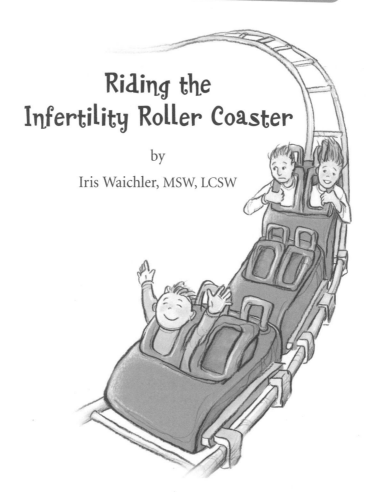

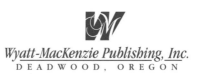
Wyatt-MacKenzie Publishing, Inc.
DEADWOOD, OREGON

Riding the Infertility Roller Coaster: A Guide to Educate and Inspire
by Iris Waichler, MSW, LCSW

Published by The Mom-Writers Publishing Cooperative
Wyatt-MacKenzie Publishing, Inc., Deadwood, OR
www.WyMacPublishing.com (541) 964-3314

Cover illustration by Kelley Cunningham, www.kelleysart.com
Index by Pueblo Indexing & Publishing Services, www.puebloindexing.com

Requests for permission or further information should be addressed to:
Wyatt-MacKenzie Publishing, 15115 Highway 36, Deadwood, Oregon 97430

Printed in the United States of America

Riding the
Infertility Roller Coaster

A Guide
to Educate & Inspire

by

Iris Waichler, MSW, LCSW

TABLE OF CONTENTS

ACKNOWLEDGEMENTS

I decided to try and write this book after spending time with many couples who had undergone some type of infertility treatment. I quickly learned that the struggles my husband and I shared had common themes with these couples. I am continuously in awe of the strength and courage displayed by the women and men that face the infertility journey.

I especially want to thank the people that agreed to be interviewed for my book. I would not have been able to write it without their help. Their honesty, their openness, and their willingness to share the most personal of stories are things I will always be grateful for. So to Sue and Howard, Ann, Todd and Eliza, and Kate and Eric, you have my eternal gratitude. I had decided that, if I couldn't find people who were willing to be interviewed, I would not go ahead with this project. Then I learned I simply had to ask, and you were all there.

I also wanted to thank Sue Gartzman and Shannon McCarthy for their editing assistance at a time it was really needed. I want to extend an additional thank you to Sue for helping me find Nancy Cleary. Without either of you this book would never have been published.

Finally, a huge debt of gratitude goes out to my husband, Steve. His editing assistance, time commitment, and writing expertise helped to make this book into something I wouldn't have imagined. He tabled other priorities in his life to help make this book happen for me. Our different approaches to the writing of the book made for some "interesting challenges" for both of us. Our shared passion regarding the importance of this subject and our intimate knowledge of infertility helped us both to stay focused on the book and what needed to be said. I also want to thank him for giving me the opportunity to balance my staying at home, being a mom, doing this book, and the counseling and speaking that I get to do. My life was forever changed, thanks to my amazing daughter Grace. I learn from her daily and her endless love, boundless humor, and wisdom stir my soul on a daily basis. My life is incredibly rich with both of you in it.

To those of you who are facing infertility I hope the information you find in this book will be helpful as you move through this difficult path. I also hope the stories and information that you find in here will give you courage, hope, and help you realize that you are not alone in your journey, whatever awaits you at the other end.

INTRODUCTION

I think it is important for you to know who I am and why I have chosen to write this book. On a personal level, I got married at age 42. My husband was 38. My mother had a long history of miscarriages. Because of her history and my age I thought having children was not possible for me. Two months after my wedding I had a miscarriage. Suddenly I realized I could get pregnant. I was shocked by the intensity of grief I felt over the loss of our child. I was surprised by the depth of my feelings and my strong desire to have a child. After talking with my husband, we began our journey to have a child through infertility treatment.

Professionally, I am a social worker. I worked in hospitals for thirteen years, primarily helping patients and families who struggled with medical, psychiatric and drug and alcohol problems. I also worked in managed care for nine years helping people connect with medical and psychiatric doctors, nurses, and therapists. Finally, I spent a year working as a claims manager for people applying for disability. I am familiar with all aspects of the healthcare system on both a personal and professional basis.

In 1988, I wrote a book called *Patient Power: How to Have a Say During Your Hospital Stay.* It was a patient advocacy book based on my observations while working in hospitals. I saw that if patients and their families had more information and knowledge, they would feel less helpless in dealing with hospitals.

My purpose in writing this book is to help people going through infertility. I want to give you the tools, knowledge, and information that can help guide you through this difficult process. I want to help you feel more empowered when asking questions or making critical decisions. I have worked with people who have had every imaginable medical or psychiatric or drug problem. Even so, I can't think of a group that is more powerless and vulnerable in the face of their treatment than people going through infertility.

I hope this book can serve as a practical guide and a one-stop source for a broad base of useful information. I will quote experts, lean on my personal and professional expertise, and the experience of many people who have been through infertility. I am hopeful that you will find infertility issues dealt with in a sensitive and thoughtful way. In the course of reading this book, you may have unanswered questions and will need to go elsewhere for further information. You will learn that those of us who struggle with infertility need to consult numerous people and resources. There is always more to learn about fighting the infertility battle, and we should be ever mindful of the growing amount of information that is available. The boundaries of possibility are constantly being stretched.

This book is meant to provide you with practical information, but it is also about people and how they make these most difficult and personal decisions. Those of us struggling with infertility need to know we are not alone. It can be a lonely, isolated feeling when you recognize that you are facing infertility. The range of emotions that can be experienced includes surprise, anger, grief, sadness, guilt, and hopelessness. Those of us facing this issue will experience a multitude of other feelings as well. Infertility is sometimes referred to as "a roller coaster ride." This metaphor exemplifies the challenging process of dealing with infertility. Infertility is a major life crisis. I will address these feelings and discuss how to cope with them throughout this book. I want to empower and educate you about the process, and give you the tools you need to negotiate this difficult journey. I wish some of these tools and information had been available to me as I faced my personal infertility journey.

In this book, you will also hear the voices of other men and women who have chosen to take this difficult journey. I think it is important to hear from both men and women. In my research for this book, men's voices were not evident in the literature. Their experiences, perspective, and feelings can be different from those of women. Their pain can also be incredibly deep. All of the people I interviewed hope that sharing their knowledge and struggles will be helpful to others struggling with infertility. These stories, told in their own words, are compelling and quite candid and will touch you. You will see how people choose to cope with infertility in different ways with different results. You may see yourself in these stories. All of us hope that you

will be able to find useful knowledge and ideas to apply to your particular situation. In my personal and professional experience, there are
common themes we all deal with in infertility, and these themes will be
revealed in the stories and discussed in the chapters ahead.

Let me introduce you to some of the people you will meet in
this book. Their stories will be more fully told in future chapters, but
here are brief sketches of their struggles with infertility. If any of the
technical terms are not familiar to you, there are detailed definitions in
the glossary in Chapter 21. I have changed people's names at their
request to protect and respect their privacy. Their generosity in opening up about the most personal and intimate of issues was greatly
appreciated by me. I hope you will feel the same way as you read this
book. Here is a brief introduction to the people and their stories of
struggling with infertility.

ELIZA AND TODD

Eliza, an account director, was twenty-seven years old when she started her infertility treatment in April of 1999. Her husband, Todd, is a
lawyer. He was thirty-four years old at that time. Eliza underwent
eleven intrauterine insemination treatments (IUI), and used many
injectible medications before she began in vitro fertilization (IVF) in
June 2001. She was ultimately successful and became pregnant. Their
daughter, Darcy, was born in March 2002.

SUE AND HOWARD

Sue works in marketing and was thirty-five years old when she began
treatment. Her husband, Howard, is a commodity trader and was thir-
ty-six years old. Sue went through four cycles of intrauterine insemination. They experienced two cancelled cycles of in vitro fertilization
(IVF) and completed a third cycle of IVF, which resulted in a miscarriage. Sue and Howard eventually chose to try using an egg donor
because she could not produce enough eggs or follicles. Their first try
using an egg donor failed, but their second cycle was successful. They
traveled out of state to have this procedure done. She was forty years
old when their son Isaac was born in January 2001.

ANN AND MARK

Ann, a psychologist, was thirty-four years old when she got married. She had always had irregular periods and anticipated that getting pregnant would be very difficult. Her husband, Mark, is a consultant, and he was forty-two years old with two children from a previous marriage. Ann began treatment at thirty-five and got pregnant within a few months but miscarried. Subsequently, she underwent many years of additional treatment, pursuing a variety of techniques, including surgeries. Eventually, her husband was tested, and Mark was diagnosed with fertility problems as well. Finally, Mark became seriously ill and they decided to stop treatment and remain childless. Mark's illness was a catalyst for making this decision sooner, but they both felt they would have chosen this outcome eventually.

KATE AND ERIC

Kate, an attorney, was forty-one years old when she got married and knew that her chances of getting pregnant were not good. Her husband, Eric, was forty-three years old and a computer programmer. They waited a year to begin infertility treatment and did one cycle of in vitro fertilization (IVF). Kate produced only a small number of follicles and only three to four eggs in that cycle. She also had a bad reaction to the medications used. A second medical opinion confirmed she was not a good candidate for having a child on her own. She and her husband agreed they would adopt a child. Their daughter, Leah, was adopted from China on November 22, 1998. Leah was ten months old at the time of her adoption.

IRIS AND STEVE

My husband and I also got married and began our infertility treatment later in life. Despite our early pregnancy, our doctor advised us that most infertility treatments would be ineffective because of my age. We did a lot of research, which confirmed what he told us, and we chose not to get a second opinion. He advised us that our best chance was to use an egg donor and that other treatment alternatives would have a low likelihood of success. We all agreed the goal was for me to get pregnant and deliver a healthy baby as quickly as possible. We got on an egg donor list and waited nine months. Our first donor got pregnant right before we were to begin treatment, so we had to start over and find another donor. Our first embryo transfer failed. Our second and final attempt (with the last of our embryos) was successful. Our daughter, Grace, was born in July of 2000.

You will hear all of our stories in greater detail later in the book. I am in awe of the courage and tenacity I have seen in the people who have gone through infertility treatment. I have had the good fortune to meet and get to know some incredible people. I think you will be in awe, too, and hopefully hearing from them will help you to move in the direction that is right for you.

My husband and I are extremely lucky to have our daughter, Grace. Steve was forty-two years old, and I was 45 years old when she was born. I will describe many of our experiences in this book. Your experiences will not necessarily be the same as mine. I hope that by sharing what shaped my thoughts and feelings, I can give you useful information to confront your own issues in this struggle. Infertility is a difficult journey, but you are not alone. There are many outcomes, and every journey is different. I hope the information in this book can empower you in making difficult decisions, and that these stories can help you to find your own way through the ups and downs of your infertility journey.

CHAPTER 1
WHAT IS INFERTILITY?

It is important to have a simple definition of what we mean by infertility. Generally, if a woman has actively engaged in unprotected sex for a year or more, and has been unsuccessful in getting pregnant or delivering a baby, then she has an infertility problem. For a man, the definition would be his inability to get a woman pregnant in the same time frame. These simple definitions are a useful starting point, but truly understanding infertility is much more complex.

Perhaps, the best way to define infertility is to look closely at how it impacts our lives. It is difficult for people who have never experienced infertility to understand just how devastating it can be. It is incredible, but infertility affects six million people in the United States, and cuts across all socioeconomic groups and professions. Chances are some of your friends, neighbors, and family are impacted by this problem. Infertility is often an unspoken crisis in life, going on around us without our knowing about it. I remember when I had a miscarriage and word slowly got out. Countless people came up to me and shared their personal stories about miscarriages. I began to feel like everybody had had this experience at some point in life.

After my miscarriage, my husband and I were at a family function and his elderly aunt came over to speak with him. She was in her eighties, and they were close and had seen each other frequently over the years. She revealed to him that she had endured nine miscarriages during her last marriage. She and her husband had both been married before, and both of them had children from their previous marriages. But they really wanted children together, yet it was not to be. Sharing this information forty years later was so painful for her that she had to excuse herself and go to the ladies room to regain her composure. Later, she came over to me and gave me a big hug.

Three things were striking to us about her story. First, we were surprised by the fact that few in the family had been aware of her struggle with infertility before that day. Second, we were struck by how vivid those memories and feelings were for her, even forty years later.

Finally, it was an early realization for me that, even when you have a child, trying again and experiencing infertility (secondary infertility) can be incredibly painful.

Secondary infertility is an important and often overlooked part of the story of infertility. This occurs when people have been successful in having children and then are unable to conceive another child. This can happen for a variety of reasons, and can also be an extremely painful experience. Friends and family may not respond in an empathetic way because they know there are already children, and even medical professionals can downplay the problem. Often, there is a lack of understanding about how difficult it is to lose the ability to have children. But these feelings of loss, sadness, and grief can be as intense as the feelings of those people who are unable to conceive any children. There can be a multitude of reasons why pregnancy is not possible. Those of us who are lucky enough to conceive a child automatically assume that we can do it again when we want to. The realization that this will not happen can be devastating. Secondary infertility is a phenomenon that is becoming more seriously recognized and acknowledged by the medical and psychological communities.

Thinking about our concepts of family can help put the feelings of loss connected with infertility into perspective. Most people grow up with the expectation that they will eventually get married and have children. When we think about the future, most of us imagine being parents and having children. We often assume that when we are ready to have a baby, it will just happen. This expectation is a message given to us by society and our parents and other family members. At times, there are even cultural and religious traditions urging us to procreate.

On a number of occasions, I have heard Catholic newlyweds describe how their families continually ask them: "When are you going to start a family?" These pressures can become a real source of stress for people. One of the couples I spoke with chose to remain childless after numerous attempts to have children failed. They were both comfortable with this decision. Even after they explained this to family members, however, they were told: "Are you sure this is what you want? Maybe you just need more time to think about it." Often, we feel that if we don't fulfill the expectations of others, they may perceive that there is something wrong with us. These subtle and not so subtle messages place pressures on us, and people experiencing infertility can feel an enormous urgency to meet these expectations.

We are all painfully aware of the "biological clock" that ticks in women as they age. The media has latched onto this concept over the years, and made it a popular image. My husband recently showed me an article that cited the percentage of American women ages forty to forty-four that are mothers. He made me guess the number. My guess wasn't even close to the numbers cited in the article. What would you guess? The article said that the number was 81%, which was down from 90% in 1980. I was really surprised by how high these numbers were. It made it clear to me how strong the urge to have children is for many women. The numbers demonstrated that this need to be a mother cuts across all socioeconomic, religious, and ethnic groups. In many women, the need to have a child is a deep, biological urge that, at times, even becomes a spiritual need. This is a basic part of human nature, but is especially true for women.

LOSS

When we address the impact of infertility we cannot overemphasize the notion of loss. It is important to understand the scope of the losses associated with infertility when we are exploring its definition. The issue of loss is one of the core consequences of infertility. In her book, *Taking Charge of Infertility*, Patricia Irwin Johnston, a noted expert on infertility, takes a close look at the series of losses that people encounter as they travel through the journey of infertility. I think it is valuable to review these losses. It is the first step in understanding how to cope with them. Ms. Johnston identifies six major areas of loss. They include the following:

Control over many aspects of life.
>Individual genetic continuity linking past and future.
>The joint conception of a child with one's life partner.
>The physical satisfactions of pregnancy and birth.
>The emotional gratifications of pregnancy and birth.
>The opportunity to parent.(1)

She goes on to describe these areas in greater detail. "Loss of control" was one area that jumped out at me immediately when I was thinking about the repercussions of infertility. These feelings begin from the moment we learn that we cannot have a child how and when we want to, and they often continue throughout our treatment period. One of my inspirations for writing this book was a lecture I heard by Naomi Wolf, a leading feminist. She was speaking about a book she had written, and her anger over a horrible experience she had in the hospital when her baby was born. She believed her doctors were forcing her to have a cesarean section when she did not want it. She said they would not hear what she had to say about it. She described feeling angry and helpless. I started thinking about the feelings of impotence those of us who undergo infertility treatment often feel when dealing with medical professionals.

Deciphering the best treatment options can be an extremely complex and frustrating process. In her book, *Infertility and Identity*, Lara Deveraux points out that: "40% of all cases of infertility are due to the combined problems of both partners."(2) She further states that in "5% to 10% of the couples who receive standardized testing nothing was wrong with either partner and the diagnosis was "unexplained infertility."(3) This is a huge source of frustration for couples who are trying to determine what treatment options are available to them. Often, finding effective treatment options can involve trial and error in these instances, because protocols are less defined when no diagnosis is apparent.

Even when we have an accurate diagnosis, the feeling of "loss of control" frequently stays with us throughout our prescribed treatment. When I first began my infertility treatment I remember a conversation I had with our nurse. In a matter-of-fact way I had told her we were planning to go on a trip at a certain time, so she would know how to plan our upcoming treatment. I heard her laugh loudly, and I think she almost dropped the telephone. She advised me that from that moment on I should throw out the notion of planning anything. That was when it first hit me that my life was not my own anymore, and that if we were going to be successful at having a baby, everything was out of my hands and totally out of my control.

I was at the mercy of doctors, nurses, and lab technicians. Often, in infertility treatment, there are people you don't know telling you what to do, how to do it, and when to do it. My husband and I did not have to explain to our doctor how and when we had sex, but many people do have to discuss this. We did not have our doctor telling us when to have sex, but this happens. Many people going through infertility are forced to share the most intimate aspects of their lives with a number of people they don't even know well. This loss of privacy can seem like an invasion of personal space, and a surrendering of control. Of course, this is all done with the ultimate goal of achieving pregnancy and a healthy baby. I did not experience the loss of control of my mood due to medications, though this is also quite common. Many women struggle with feelings they cannot explain and do things they don't mean to because of all the stress, anxiety, or medications that come with infertility treatment.

I am one of those people who like control and need to plan. When I was working I would have a list on my desk, and by the end of the day everything was checked off. The surrendering of control was a huge adjustment for me. It was a leap of faith. I had to throw out my checklist and, worse yet, have somebody else write it. I realized later that I did have more control than I thought. However, it never felt that way during my infertility treatment. I will explain how to take some of this control back in later chapters. You can find examples of this in Chapters 2 and 3.

Surprisingly, for those of us who are lucky enough to get pregnant, these feelings of powerlessness often remain with us throughout our entire pregnancy. Most of us just can't bring ourselves to believe that we are going to have a healthy baby until we see and hold our child. We find ourselves waiting for something else that is unexpected and unplanned to occur. "Loss of control" is one of the themes I heard over and over again from virtually everybody who underwent some type of infertility treatment successfully. I will address the dynamic of these feelings in pregnancy in much more detail in Chapter 13, Pregnant at Last.

GENETICS

Genetic continuity is another issue that often emerges in infertility treatment. Our concepts of family are deeply tied to genetics. This connection has strong familial and cultural roots. Many people feel it is their duty to continue their family genetic line from generation to generation. "The family name must go on," is one common way this is expressed. The issue of genetic continuity surrounds us in many of the spoken and unspoken messages we are given. This issue is deeply embedded in our thinking and challenges many people struggling with infertility.

For people who feel it is their duty to continue the genetics of their family, infertility can be especially devastating. Ann, one of the people I interviewed for my book, addressed this issue quite eloquently. "My parents escaped the Holocaust and lost most of their family," she told me. She had always felt that her parents believed it was critical for her to have children because of this history. When she examined her own feelings about not being able to have children, she found this part of it particularly difficult. "To continue the family line was very important to me," she said, "and I just assumed it was difficult for my parents." When people feel strongly about genetic continuity, the dilemma of infertility can feel even more overwhelming.

Many of us don't want to disappoint family members, but often we don't talk with them about the issue of genetic continuity, either. If you feel comfortable doing it, it can be important to discuss this with your family. Bringing it out in the open at least provides some sense of certainty about what everybody thinks and feels. You may be surprised at the reaction, as Ann was. She learned her parents were comfortable with whatever choices she made regarding children. She never would have known this if she had not discussed it with them. Their reaction was not what she anticipated. I describe Ann's story in much more detail in Chapter 10, Making the Choice to Live Childfree.

Most of us dream of having a child some day and pick a partner with qualities and traits we hope to impart to our children. Many people try to imagine how their unborn child will resemble family members or what family personality traits will emerge. It is hard for many of us to let go of this dream of conceiving a child together, with both parents' genetics commingled. But more and more people are forfeiting this dream in order to have a child in other ways. But even after making this choice, many people remain very focused on the genetics of their child. Some people even come to see it as an opportunity. I have heard many people say they are not particularly happy with their genetics and do not want to pass any potential health problems on to their unborn children. People with a strong family history of cancer, for example, often have fears about passing on a predisposition to their potential offspring.

Using an egg or sperm donor or pursuing adoption can even be perceived by some people as an opportunity to select for improved genetics. The campus newspapers at Ivy League schools are full of ads from couples seeking "high potential" donors. They can list targets for test scores, subject majors, sports aptitude, height, weight, and coloration—even extra-curricular interests. These potential parents are just as wrapped up as other parents in imagining their future child, but of course, there are no guarantees regarding our genetic makeup.

Newborn babies are unpredictably unique, and their combination of genetics is like a kind of alchemy. If you use a sperm or egg donor, or you opt to adopt a child, you are given information about the genetic parent. Some people feel this situation gives them more genetic choice and control. However, you cannot always be certain that all the information you have been given is totally accurate, or that it is predictive. Some genetic traits skip generations, and others emerge as a result of combining the genes from two parents. Accuracy of genetic history can be a particularly important issue with international adoptions. In some countries the legal requirements governing the documentation of the adoptive child differ from those in the United States. This varies greatly from country to country. Chapter 9 reviews these issues relating to adoption.

Some people approach these questions in another way. They believe that children's personalities can be shaped through the environmental and behavioral influences of the parents rather than genetics. This is the other side of the often-posed question of "nature vs. nurture." The psychological community seems to agree that a child is born with certain traits or temperament, such as adaptability or sensitivity. These traits impact how the child experiences his or her sense of self. The nurture side of the equation suggests that the type of interplay a parent has with a child can impact how these traits emerge. Many parents that do not share genetics with their children are comforted by this idea. They believe that they can still influence the development of their child in many ways, regardless of their genetic make-up.

PARENTING AS A RITE OF PASSAGE

Many women feel that they are not complete unless they are able to become pregnant and have a child. The infertility struggle forces us to look deep inside ourselves and gain a better understanding of how we cope with major life obstacles and who we are as people. Sue, another interviewee, told me: "I always listened to a lot of other people talk about how it...made them question their worth as a woman...like they weren't a complete person because of infertility. I never felt that way. I think it made me...view myself as a more assertive, aggressive person. That was the part of me that I had to look at and question—yes, my ability to assert myself. That was the heart of myself and my ability to change."

The author Patricia Johnston also points out: "Many people see the loss of pregnancy as belonging entirely to women, but this is not true. Though physical changes and challenges of pregnancy and birth are experienced by women alone, producing a child...is the ultimate rite of passage for both men and women—the final mark of reaching adulthood."(4) The point she makes is important: men are significantly impacted by their partners' pregnancies and having children. This is often overlooked. The inability of his partner to have a child can also be devastating for the man. Todd, one husband I interviewed, shared his feelings about infertility treatment. He stated: "There were people who just didn't realize what a sensitive topic it was, and the fact that we were trying it and it didn't happen for a long time was really personally difficult." Many men have a feeling of helplessness. There can be a sense of frustration, because they want to help in any way they can, but they may not be certain how to do this.

Sometimes, doctors don't take the time to give information to men, or they don't include them in all the treatment discussions they have with their partners. The focus of infertility treatment is often on women. Doctors may also assume the man has a greater understanding of what is going on, of the medical issues or treatment, than he does. In an interview with Sue's husband, Howard, he described the moment when a doctor told him that she had endometriosis. The doctor never explained what this meant. Howard's reaction was: "What's that? Is it going to kill her?" He told me he "raced to the library" to find out what this meant. The doctor came out later and told him: "I am going to scrape her out." Howard, a terrified husband, didn't understand and he asked himself: "Is it eating her away?" You will hear directly from the men I interviewed about how infertility issues impacted them. There are both similarities and differences between how men and women react during this struggle.

Patricia Johnston makes reference to "the emotional gratification of a shared pregnancy" on her list of losses. People imagine how pregnancy will impact their relationship with their partner. There are lots of books and classes to prepare us for this experience. Friends and family are often eager to offer advice, whether we ask for it or not. We see idealized versions of pregnancy everywhere in the print and TV media. During my interview with Ann, she shared the feelings she had when she began to realize she was infertile. She told me, "I had a man who I wanted to spend my life with and I was running out of time. I was mad at my body—like a lot of people. I finally was in a good situation where I felt this was a good relationship to bring children into and all I had was two step-children." While Mark had children from a previous marriage, if Ann's fertility treatment failed, they wouldn't share the experience of a pregnancy and birth of their own baby. They would also miss the experience of parenting a young child together. Many people feel these experiences are vital to fulfilling the potential of a relationship, and creating the strong, mutual identity shared in a family.

In my research, I found that one of the best perspectives on the impact of infertility on relationships came from a book called *The Fertility Book* by Richard Marrs, M.D., Lisa Friedman-Bloch and Kathy Kirtland Silverman. In this book the authors write, "The way you define infertility is it grows out of the way it impacts your personality. Each of us has come to where we are with different expectations for your life. Reach down, deep inside yourself and find what being infertile means in relation to these life goals... You and your partner should understand each other's answers thoroughly."(5) Infertility can seem to drive a wedge into some relationships. Sorting out its impacts on our personalities and expectations can take a real commitment to mutual exploration as a couple. It's not always easy to understand the perspective of your partner and find shared goals, when you're struggling with infertility. There are costs to pay—financial, physical, and emotional—that can tax even the most solid relationships. Both partners need to know how the other feels and decisions need to be shared.

INFORMATION, TECHNOLOGY, AND INFERTILITY

Today there are many places to go to learn about infertility, and I believe this is a good thing. It is being talked about quite openly on television, and in newspapers and magazines. Society in general is much more open today about infertility issues, and we recognize that more people are choosing to have children later in their lives. Topics that were taboo in the past are openly discussed today. We would never have encountered an interview with a couple and their surrogate five years ago. Today, we see stories about the phenomenon of older and older women having babies on a regular basis.

When I began to do research for my book, I went on the Internet and punched in infertility. There were over 15,000 possible sites that I could explore. The available information is growing on a steady basis, and I hope this trend continues. But you do need to be cautious about what you read and the information that is given to you. This is especially true in regard to the Internet. People are well aware that infertility is a very painful situation and some may try to take advantage of people coping with this problem. Be sure you check any information you are given with an appropriate professional or a trusted and knowledgeable confidant.

The infertility treatment options available to us today are greater than ever before. We can have children through surrogacy, sperm donation, egg or embryo donation, and adoption (foreign and domestic). Some of these treatment options are quite controversial and some people find their religious or ethical belief systems challenged by these new possibilities. Medicine and science have joined together to offer us more treatment options, and the rate of success is rising. There are new medications available to enhance our abilities to produce eggs and sperm, and to improve their quality. Doctors can now test for genetic abnormalities in an embryo prior to implantation. Medical research has established more successful ways to transfer these eggs and embryos to ensure a higher number of them will result in pregnancy. But as the science advances, it can challenge our ethical or religious beliefs, and often there are very personal judgements to make.

Whatever your personal belief system, you will need to understand the treatment options and how they work. In the glossary in Chapter 21 you will find definitions for many of the medical options available, including types of treatment and medications used in infertility treatment. In addition to sorting out the different types of treatment, picking the right doctor is critical to your understanding of your treatment and to its success. In the next chapter, I will explain how to pick a doctor and what questions to ask about his or her training and experience in infertility treatment. Picking the right doctor and support staff can be critical to having a successful pregnancy. The right doctor will also help you come to a thorough understanding of the ethical implications of your choice of treatment. For many people, exploring ethical issues with their doctor is critical to their personal decision-making, and this requires a special patient-doctor relationship.

My husband and I were quite amazed at how rapidly the technology changed throughout the year and a half we underwent our infertility treatment. I discussed this with my doctor, and he told me that there seemed to be a new breakthrough happening every few months. My doctor explained to me that the success rate for our particular reproductive technique improved ten to fifteen percent from the time we initiated treatment until the time we conceived.

Recently, I heard a story on the news about a woman who had twin children born through in vitro fertilization. She had an additional embryo frozen. She decided thirteen years after the birth of her twin children to unfreeze this third embryo and try to have another child. This treatment was successful and she had a girl. At the time of her birth, they realized she was the third child of triplets. There was a difference in age of thirteen years between the first two and the third triplet. This was the first time an embryo frozen that long resulted in a healthy baby. It was an incredible story. The mother laughed and said her older girls had a hard time explaining to their friends that this new sister was a triplet, too.

I thought this was a great example of the complexity of infertility treatment. It illustrates some of the interesting challenges successful treatment can bring to us as parents, siblings, and families. I also mention this example because it is important that you can speak frankly with your doctor about your treatment wishes and their potential consequences. Your doctor needs to have a good understanding of the current available reproductive technology, and what type of treatment offers you the best chance at conception and fulfilling your treatment needs. Your doctor should also have some experience performing the latest infertility treatment methods. There is no substitute for experience with patients, and doctors actively using a variety of treatment techniques have a greater understanding of the efficacy and ramifications of the treatments for different individuals. The professional competence of your doctor is critical, but the best practitioners are also good listeners and communicators.

A good fertility practice will help you explore the personal and ethical implications of your treatment options, but they will also leave you to decide what treatment to pursue based on your own beliefs. Your doctor should be willing to explore these issues with you before a final decision is made on what treatment option to pursue. My husband and I were lucky. We found a doctor who was willing to spend a lot of time getting to know us. He was also highly experienced. In the end, we skipped a lot of potential treatment options because of my age and our circumstances. Our doctor was wise enough and honest enough with us that we knew not to try infertility techniques that had little or no hope of working. Our doctor also took to the time to find out who we were and what we really wanted.

INFERTILITY AS A CRISIS

Dealing with infertility and its various medical treatments can be an ongoing challenge. Barbara Eck Manning is a pioneer nurse who helped begin a national organization, RESOLVE, which works for advocacy and education on behalf of people with infertility issues. She has done extensive writing around infertility issues and addresses the issue of infertility as a crisis in her book, *Guide for the Childless Couple.* In this book she quotes Gerald Caplan's definition of a crisis. He states a crisis is "a stressful event that poses a problem that is unsolvable in the immediate future. The problem overtaxes the existing resources of the persons involved because it is beyond traditional problem solving methods. The problem is perceived as a threat to important life goals of the persons involved. Finally, it reawakens unsolved problems from both the near and distant past."(6) This really rang true for me as I read it. It is a perfect description of what happens to people in the midst of the infertility struggle.

Infertility can become an all-consuming crisis that you must live with on a daily basis. During treatment, the need to give yourself injections, to go for blood work, or to undergo endless tests are daily reminders that your body is not functioning the way you want it to. When I was interviewing Eliza for this book, she expressed the idea that seeking infertility treatment can become an all-consuming process. She told me: "It becomes addictive. It really becomes addictive. This doesn't work and let me move on to the next infertility treatment. The doctor told us the odds were in our favor. We kept going." Anyone who has had to face infertility treatment understands the feeling of being stuck. Infertility becomes an all-consuming aspect of life, tied to everything that we do.

I mentioned earlier that the number of treatment options available to us is growing at an astonishing rate. The histories of the people that I interviewed suggest only a small number of the options that are available to us today. Once we are faced with the knowledge we are infertile, we can choose to explore a great number of treatment options. Many people begin by trying to have their own child, which can be pursued in many ways. Each treatment option has a different likelihood of success in each situation. I strongly encourage everyone going through infertility to speak at length with your doctor about the specific treatment opportunities that would be the best match for you and your individual medical situation. You and your doctor share the goal of having a successful pregnancy and a healthy baby. Your doctor will likely be encouraging, and it is common to try a sequence of treatments over time in order to fulfill this goal. You should have a clear understanding with your doctor about your likely success rate for each type of treatment, and how long each option might need to be pursued.

Issues around disclosure are another way that infertility can seem like a crisis. What we communicate, how we communicate, and when we communicate can seem impossibly complicated. Ann's delayed communication with her parents or Todd's characterization of others as "insensitive" provide classic examples of how disclosure and its issues can linger and remain unresolved. In upcoming chapters you will learn what to say to family and friends who do not seem sensitive to your individual situation. You will hopefully benefit from the experience and words of the people I interviewed. We will look at issues of disclosure; how to build a support network; and balancing life, treatment, and work.

The personal challenges we face do not necessarily end, even if we succeed in getting pregnant and having a baby. As I highlighted earlier, pregnancy after infertility can be extremely stressful, and seem to perpetuate a state of crisis. Anxiety about completing the pregnancy and having a healthy baby is common. Many older women have to deal with additional medical complications in pregnancy and birth due to their age. These factors can compound the natural worries we have about pregnancy and delivery. Even after we deliver a healthy baby, parenting a newborn is also very demanding. Sleep deprivation is common, and being a new parent is never easy. Some of us have started our infertility journey later in life and will become parents at an older age. Older parents face unique challenges that are often not addressed in the literature. I felt it was imperative to address pregnancy after infertility, parenting after infertility, and being an older parent in this book. My research showed that these areas received little attention.

Successful infertility treatment can perpetuate disclosure issues, too. Depending upon how our children are conceived, disclosure issues can continue long after they are born. These issues can include disclosure about genetics to family and friends, and social disclosure within our wider world of acquaintances. How much to tell people and when to tell them can be challenging questions to answer, particularly as our children grow up. Ultimately, these questions involve disclosure to the children, too, and how to eventually give them control of this disclosure themselves. I will spend some time looking at all these challenges in greater detail in Chapter 17. Listing them here illustrates how the crisis of infertility can continue even when treatment is successful.

When treatment is not successful, the feeling of being in perpetual crisis can be heightened. There may always be one more option to try, no matter how slim its chances, and deciding to stop treatment can be particularly difficult. It is important to maintain hope while you are undergoing treatment, but it is equally important to be realistic about your chances of achieving the goal of a healthy birth. Making the decision to stop treatment is very difficult, and postponing this decision is a common source of ongoing crisis in infertility. If you decide that delivering a baby is not an achievable goal for you, then other options, including adoption, surrogacy, or choosing to live a life without a child are viable choices that you can make and should explore.

I will examine each of these options in greater detail later in the book. They all come with their own complex set of personal decisions. Chapter 9 will explore questions surrounding adoption. Is it right for you? When should you consider adoption, and where should you go to find a child? What process will you have to go through to become an adoptive parent? Chapter 8 looks into the complicated issues associated with surrogacy, and having someone else carry and deliver your baby. How do you find and choose a surrogate? What legal questions need to be addressed with your surrogate? What questions should you ask yourself about whether this is the right treatment option for you? How do you decide what role the surrogate will play in your child's future life? Each of these choices has profound personal implications, and every option is complex in its own way, raising challenging questions to resolve. There is no "right" answer and making these challenging decisions requires a lot of study and soul-searching.

I also want to explore the idea of choosing not to have children, which is covered in Chapter 10. This is as an option you may need to consider for yourself as you go through your journey. My husband and I talked about this during my treatment, and it informed some of the choices we made. I will explore the issue of when to take a look at this option and what questions to ask to determine if this decision is right for you and your partner. I will also examine ways to address this issue with family and friends. Deciding to end your pursuit of parenthood is often not the end of the infertility journey, though. Remaining childless can profoundly impact our sense of self, of continuity, and of purpose for the rest of our lives. Chapter 19 looks at the impacts of different fertility outcomes on the life of a couple, and explores how couples can renew themselves to move forward. Whatever the outcome of our struggles, infertility tends to stay with us and become part of our experience and who we are.

In this chapter we have looked at defining infertility and its strong impact on all areas of our lives. The desire to have a family and to maintain its continuity runs deep in many of us. That is part of the reason the problem of infertility cuts so deeply into our lives. The purpose of this book is to empower you so that you will have some additional skills and knowledge to help you navigate the inevitable hurdles that go along with infertility. You will hear the people I've interviewed speak about these challenges and decisions, and how they weighed their options. You will also hear about some of the fears they faced alone and with their partners. You will likely face many of the same hurdles in your journey through infertility. It is a struggle that often redefines us, a rite of passage where we can't always chose the outcome. Always remember you are not alone, and that others are making this journey, too. Finding support in others is often important, wherever your journey leads. Every possible outcome happens to many other people. Sharing our experiences with others often helps us find our own individual resolution in the struggle of dealing with infertility.

CHAPTER 2
FINDING YOUR DOCTOR

One of the most important tasks when you begin your infertility treatment is finding the right doctor. I believe there are two critical components to finding the right doctor and having a good doctor-patient relationship. First, the doctor's medical knowledge and skill are imperative to being successful at helping you become pregnant. Secondly, you need to feel comfortable talking to your doctor. You will have countless questions and concerns that arise as you venture into this unknown territory and you will need to consult closely with your doctor. Ultimately, your doctor should be able to help you understand and assess the best treatment options in your particular case, and he or she should leave the final choice of treatment up to you. Once you make this choice, your doctor must be capable of executing the chosen treatment competently.

Many of us have had the same internist or obstetrician for many years and have developed a long and strong relationship with him or her. Once you learn that infertility is an issue, you need to be referred to a reproductive endocrinologist (RE). Sometimes you need to be proactive about getting this referral. Make sure your internist or obstetrician/gynecologist is someone who can recognize when you need to see a specialist. Don't wait for him or her to make the referral when you feel a referral to a specialist is needed. Be proactive and discuss this with your doctor. Don't wait for him or her to bring it up.

In my interview with Eliza, she told me about some difficulties she had with her doctor. She said: "Our experience sort of proved that you really have to have a doctor that you emotionally click with. My gynecologist had me take my temperature every day and told me: 'You don't have a problem; let's check your husband.' And she sent him to the nastiest urologist on the planet. All he wanted to do was operate." Bad experiences with doctors are an indication that you need to make a change. Good communication is essential, and if your doctor won't listen to your concerns, then a change is needed. As Eliza said, "clicking" with your doctor is important. Good doctors will help you understand your diagnosis and treatment options and be open to your questions. They will also try to understand who you are and what treatment options you prefer.

Getting a referral for a reproductive endocrinologist is a first step. This will probably be a new person, at a time when you are already very anxious about taking this next step. Be sure to assess your new doctor carefully before beginning treatment. There are guidelines you can use to make sure you find the right doctor for you. A lot of the success in infertility treatment is based on the doctor's ability to interpret blood tests, hormone levels, and a host of other tests. You should assess your doctor's experience by asking what reproductive methods he has used and how many patients he has treated successfully. You should also assess his communication skills and availability. The other crucial component is the doctor's support staff. You should assess the general competency of the practice or clinic and also the level of engagement they have with you as a patient. Be sure and ask specifically about their success rates for the procedures you may have. Assessing all these components is critical in making an informed choice. Ultimately, you should also "click," and your choice of doctor and clinic should feel right.

The sensitivity of doctors and staff can be an important part of effective treatment. Eliza described another painful episode she had when she went in for a sonogram and had a bad experience with the technician. "My doctor told me I had to have a sonogram tomorrow and that was when the heartbeat stopped," Eliza said. "I had been staring at the screen and the technician refused to tell me what was going on. I had seen enough sonograms to know what was going on. She left the probe in me with my grandmother holding it. And then, when my gynecologist found out that there was a problem, she refused to reschedule anything with me because she was going on vacation." In contrast, Eliza said: "My fertility doctor, who I called after the sonogram, said come over here immediately, and she determined the pregnancy was over. She was supposed to go on vacation the next day. She cancelled her vacation for me. I think that sums up: if you are not clicking with you doctor get rid of them."

Sue described how she experienced problems with her doctor's support staff. She explained: "They were really busy and some things fell through the cracks. At one point they told me I was pregnant and I really wasn't. They did the HCG test at a point when the drug was still in my body and for a whole weekend we thought I was pregnant, and then two days later they redid the test and found out I wasn't. That was really hard for us and we lost a lot of faith in our clinic."

Howard added, "I think what it boils down to is that they get so busy they get insensitive, it's like anyone."

In sharing his story with me, Eric talked about something that stuck with him in his discussion with their doctor. He also had advice for others going to find a doctor and speaking with them for the first time. "When you are talking to the doctor about your chances," he said, "[ask about] the results…I think in our case, what you want to [do is]…try to pin them down to be more specific. What I mean is in the sense that for patients in the age range of 40-45 the success rate is x. What he didn't say is the success rate of x was in the 40-41 year old range and the results for women 42-45 were different…I was not sure about our particular doctor, looking back, some of the questions I had or some of the concerns I had and I asked him about…he would just brush them off. I would have felt better about myself if I [had been] a more savvy customer."

Eric's story illustrates the importance of talking with your doctor about success rates, and making sure that they clearly correspond to the appropriate statistics for your specific age and diagnosis. This information is critically important when assessing different types of infertility treatment with your doctor. Make sure your doctor is providing you with transparent and accurate information that is specific to you. Sometimes asking questions is the best way to get to an accurate correspondence of the information with your individual case. As Eric says, "Be savvy."

STORIES FROM THE TRENCHES

My personal experience with doctors was mixed. I knew about a particular reproductive endocrinologist from my work in a hospital. He was the one I wanted to work with when I learned I was infertile. I met with him and knew immediately he was the right doctor for me. He asked the right questions and gave me honest answers about what my options were. He also spent some time trying to understand what I wanted. I brought my husband in to meet him before we went any farther in my treatment. I thought it was crucial my husband also felt comfortable with him. I also knew my husband was not particularly fond of any doctors. This doctor spent two hours with me and my husband. He answered all of Steve's questions and put him totally at ease. We knew we could contact him any time with any further questions, and he was in tune with our emotional and medical needs. He carefully explained everything to us every step of the way. He won my husband over immediately.

Later, there was a political and financial upheaval at our clinic—and at a very crucial moment in my treatment. I learned that my doctor was no longer allowed to treat me. We were told that he was "gone," but no one would tell us where he went. I asked who would be replacing him, and they gave me the name of another doctor with whom I was familiar. I asked when I could call her to discuss my case and was told she was not available to do that. I knew immediately I did not want to work with her and informed the clinic. They then referred me to the doctor who was now the head of the clinic.

Much later, we learned that our clinic was going into bankruptcy. They had expanded too rapidly. In the interim they were borrowing against their receivables and buying time till they could launch an IPO and "get rich quick." Their focus was obviously not on medicine, and our doctor, along with some of his best colleagues, was forced to cut costs. There was apparently a lawsuit, which reinstated them briefly, and we were told he would be "coming back." But before that happened, the clinic played its trump card and cancelled his malpractice insurance. The clinic had excellent medical practices—and they seemed to continue throughout this ordeal—but the whole episode was distracting and added stress. In the end, we lost some of our "upfront" money in the bankruptcy, too.

Now I was assigned to the head of the clinic and had to see him for a surgical procedure. We scheduled a pre-arranged phone consultation, but then had to wait forty-five minutes on hold. When the doctor finally got on the phone, it was clear that he had never even bothered to open my chart. I was furious. It was clear he had no idea who I was. I felt like a widget on an assembly line. Later, the time came for my procedure, and that was our first meeting. I nicknamed him the "Lone Ranger" because he was wearing his surgical mask when he came in and kept it on the whole time. He came into the surgical room and slapped me on the back, telling me, "It is a good day to get pregnant." He did the fifteen minute procedure without explaining anything to us. When he was done, he simply walked out of the room. I nervously asked my husband to confirm for me that he actually did anything. Later, my husband I agreed this was someone we would not work with again, and, in fact, we did make a switch soon after that.

Ann also shared her doctor experiences with me. "I had a really good doctor," she said. "I had a lot of confidence in him, and then at a certain point, I didn't think he had any new ideas. That's when we made the change. The new doctor was an RE. The thing that was the worst part of that practice was the support staff. They were a bunch of very unempathic people who—you just had the feeling—didn't get it and were busy filing their nails. I couldn't reach my doctor. I had to go through them and they weren't very good. If I really needed to talk with my doctor, I couldn't get him and that made me crazy! I would be at work waiting to get information, and they would not call. The things he wanted us to do did not feel right. I went to this other doctor who had been the main guy for years. He was probably eighty years old and his support staff were honeys. There weren't piles of people waiting to see him. I could reach him directly. That was great. I had nothing left in terms of pregnancies, but I felt his support. The trust was there. He actually read my file. When I went to see him, he knew who I was. That was important to me."

Ann and I talked some more about doctors, and I think she put it really well when I asked her what advice she would give others about choosing a doctor. She told me: "Try to figure out what is most important to you. There are a lot of good doctors out there. Ask about their success rates. Personally, I think that what is more important is [knowing whether you] are... the kind of person that wants to have the doctor who has had the most success... (I initially went to the doctor who seemed the most skilled), or do you use somebody, as I later did, that has...some human beings there to respect your needs? That has to be a part of the practice. Also look at how they organize their practice. Are they present in terms of when they have their IVF's? Is there some flexibility there?"

I think Ann put it eloquently. We often don't realize that we do have options when we are seeing a doctor. In the descriptions above, we all outlined examples of what we felt were good and bad medical treatment. You will know it in your heart and in your gut. Both Ann and I gave you an example of knowing we were not getting the medical attention we felt we needed and deserved, and we made a switch with a very positive outcome. You do not need to feel you are in a position where you are stuck with someone, especially at a time in your life when having trust in your doctor is absolutely imperative. You can turn your vulnerability around and recognize you have more power than you realize.

Sue and Howard were also eager to share advice about working with doctors and their support staff. Sue recommended: "Talk to other people and find out their horror stories. I didn't do it, but now, having heard so many war stories, that is my suggestion."

Howard quickly added: "In talking to the doctor—when they are talking to you about the whole process and everything—if you don't understand them, stop them and ask them, because so many times people say: 'Uh huh, OK.' And then your spouse doesn't know what they were talking about either. This is especially true for the first interview, since they will take more time then, because they want you as a customer. I would press them for details about everything you don't understand. Also, it turns out the person you talk to the most is the nurse so you should meet him or her."

Kate also talked with me about her doctor recollections. She told me: "I switched and took all of my records to another doctor to get a second opinion. You really have to know the nature of it is very chemical, it is blood work, ultrasounds, and somewhat of a guessing game and timing. My one doctor never even touched me to examine me. I have had friends of mine that talk about what you really want to know is what the lab people are like. That is very critical. I felt stronger after I went to the second doctor that his lab people might have been a little more competent than the first place I went."

TRANSITIONS INTO AND OUT OF TREATMENT

One thing that surprised me was my reaction when I switched from my RE back to my obstetrician. In talking with friends who underwent infertility treatment I learned that this was a common reaction. It was very hard to make the switch, even though the RE was a new doctor and my obstetrician was somebody I had worked with for many years. I actually felt a bit abandoned when I was referred back to my obstetrician. I gained a better understanding about this when I explored my feelings by talking with friends.

I realized that I had built up a real dependency on my RE and his support staff. I was going to their office many times a week, and a sense of security built up in conjunction with those regular visits. The repeated ultrasounds and heart monitor tests reassured me that my baby was safe. Also, seeing them frequently made me feel that, if something did go wrong, it would be caught immediately. Now I was being referred to a place where they told me, "We will see you in a month." A month felt like a long time to wait after I was used to seeing a doctor or nurse much more frequently. I mention this so you are aware that this is a normal reaction. Again being prepared and educated can help to normalize feelings and be a source of empowerment.

There are many reproductive endocrinologists practicing all over the United States, so there are many choices available to you. Some are good, and some are not. Some RE's have specific specialty areas so you can inquire about this. There are a number of places you can go for help in choosing a doctor. A referral from a medical professional you already know and trust is a good place to start. Also, RESOLVE, a nation-wide, non-profit organization that advocates and educates around infertility issues can be a good resource. Look in Chapter 22 for information about how to contact your local chapter of RESOLVE. They will have a list of names of specialists and their locations in your geographic area.

You should also talk to your friends and relatives. Find out if anyone knows someone with firsthand experience that you can talk to. Ask them about the quality of care they received. Think long and hard about what aspects of treatment are the most important to you. Does your partner agree with your priorities? Try to come to some common ground about your expectations for the practitioners you will be working with. We were surprised about what a fountain of information friends could be. Benefit from the experience of others. The bottom line, though, is you have to take responsibility for interviewing your practitioners, and not necessarily just take the first referral that you get.

One valuable lesson I have learned in my experience is that, if you are going to a new doctor, be sure and take any obstetric/gynecological medical records with you. You should also provide all other medical records that may be pertinent. For example, I had thyroid surgery years ago, and that information was critical in terms of looking at my infertility issues. You should provide any of your medical work ups that might relate to changes in hormones. Any previous surgeries or enzyme problems should also be discussed with your RE. This information is invaluable in cases of infertility treatment. It will give your new doctor the opportunity to make comparisons between your current medical status and past medical information. This can be especially helpful in making diagnostic judgments and treatment decisions. Try to get this information to your new doctor prior to your first appointment so he or she will have a chance to review it. This simple act may save you time and prevent you from having to undergo any unnecessary medical procedures. It will also save you money that might have been spent on unnecessary tests and procedures.

In their book, *The Fertility Book*, the authors Richard Marrs, M.D., Lisa Friedman-Bloch, and Kathy Kirtland Silverman make some very useful suggestions about what questions to ask when you are looking for a doctor and clinic. They write:

> The five most important questions to ask your doctor prior to entering any type of treatment are:
> - What is your background and training?
> - How many of these procedures do you perform annually?
> - What is your pregnancy rate per procedure?
> - What is your baby rate per procedure?
> - Who does more of these procedures annually than you and how do their success rates compare with yours?(7)

Remember statistics are often difficult to interpret and understand, and you do want to be clear when you are talking to the doctor. There is a difference between pregnancy rates and live birth rates, so be sure you get information on both of these statistics. Ask them to break down the different types of IVF procedures they do, and how many cycles they perform annually. Also get specific information on success rates for pregnancy and live births for women your age and with your diagnosis.

The Center for Disease Control puts out a booklet every few years with data on clinics throughout the country and their success rates. They look at the type of infertility treatment done and the ages of the people who have undergone the treatment. However, this data is usually a few years old. Also, when reviewing statistics on doctors and clinics, you have to keep in mind the population that they serve. Some clinics will only work with women in their twenties, so their odds of successful infertility treatments are higher, and their pregnancy data looks better. Remember to ask about the type of patients your doctor has experience working with.

If the doctor is unwilling to take the time to discuss this or does not want to answer these questions, than you may want to seek medical assistance from somebody else. You don't know how long you may be working with your reproductive endocrinologist. You hope that it will be a short time, but treatment may continue over an extended period and you want that ongoing relationship to be a strong and positive one. The support staff of your doctor is also another key ingredient of your infertility treatment experience and your potential for success. This can include the nurses, the staff members who draw your blood, the person who does your ultrasound, the receptionist, your embryologist, and the people who help interpret your lab work and test results. Ann talked about the significance of their role in her decision about choosing a doctor. I have another story that really illustrates this point.

ANOTHER TALE FROM THE TRENCHES

A friend of mine told me a story about how important sympathetic staff at the fertility clinic had been to her and her husband.

They were undergoing an IVF procedure with an egg donor, and the clinic needed a sperm sample from her husband in order to fertilize the retrieved eggs. He was "on call," and had to get up very early one morning to go provide sperm. Both his wife and the donor had already been undergoing daily treatments for a month, including countless blood draws and injections. His only previous clinical experience was providing an earlier sperm sample for analysis. Now, he found himself back in the cold, sterile room with the sink, the leather reclining chair, and the pornographic magazines and videos. He had been given a cup again and was told to be careful to provide a "clean" sample. This meant he had to wash and disinfect his hands and then use no lubricating substance that might "taint" the sample.

He went into the room and didn't come out for a very long time. He grew very uncomfortable in that room and, as much as he wanted to, he could not produce the necessary sample. The longer it took the more anxious he got, and the more impossible (and painful) the task became. "A guy masturbates a million times in his life," he said later, "but the one time you really have to do it—when the possibility of having kids depends upon it—you suddenly can't. All the pressure doesn't make it any easier."

Eventually, he emerged from the room, without a sample and terribly upset. He called his wife and she left work to come to the clinic to see what she could do to help. He felt awful because he knew all of the things his wife and their donor had undergone in their treatment to prepare for this moment. He knew all the expense that had been incurred, and that there were eggs now retrieved and waiting, with their time of viability counting down. Producing this sperm sample was the one thing he had to do to assist with treatment and he was unable to do it. This was probably their last shot at having children, so there was a lot at stake.

They went for a walk and talked a long time to try to relax him. Nothing seemed to be working. The husband was quite distraught, and they were trying to accept the worst. They spoke with the nurse and the embryologist, and explained that it didn't look like he was going to be able to produce the sperm sample they needed. The staff was incredibly empathetic. They explained that sometimes infertility treatment can be extremely difficult for men. This is rarely discussed. They told the couple that sometimes it really helps to get out of the clinic as a way to relax. They mentioned that there was a hotel up the road and encouraged the couple to think about giving it a try.

My friend and her husband were quite desperate and willing to do whatever they needed to facilitate her pregnancy. They went to the hotel with the specimen cup, and all of their hopes and dreams of being parents depended upon what happened in the next hour. Outside of the cold setting in the clinic, they were able to relax and even joke about whether they could pay for the hotel room by the hour. The end of the story is a happy one. Thanks to the wonderful suggestion of the support staff (and the help of his loving wife) he was ultimately able to produce a good sperm sample. They quickly paid their hotel bill and rushed back to the clinic in time to fertilize their eggs. They are now proud parents.

The example in this story illustrates that there is no "half way" in terms of your commitment to infertility treatment. This means the commitment from both the man and the woman. This is clearly addressed in *The Fertility Book.* Its authors note: "Treatment can also demand daily and weekly commitments of several hours during parts of your cycle. Not only will this have to be allowed for, it must take precedence over everything else in your life, including family and work related responsibilities. One missed step during a month's cycle could be the cause of a failed attempt. It's too expensive to dabble. You have to commit to your treatment 100%."(8) Infertility treatment can be highly stressful, both physically and emotionally, and my friend and her husband are a good example of the level of commitment it takes to succeed sometimes.

The Fertility Book goes on to provide this sound piece of advice: "Given [the necessary level of commitment], a factor to consider when choosing your doctor is whether the office is conveniently located relative to your home and office. If it's not, you'll have to set aside additional time to get there. Periodically, longer blocks of time may also be called for. If you're facing one of the assisted reproductive procedures, you'll have to spend several hours the day before your outpatient surgery preparing, and possibly spend several days afterwards recuperating."(9)

I can tell you from my personal experience that this is true. You may have to go to your clinic or doctor's office a lot and should also be prepared to dedicate time whenever necessary, and for as long as it takes. The timing of fertility treatments is not always predictable in advance, either.

Your doctor is going to be a critical source of information for you about timing. He or she will be one of the major components in successfully managing the progression of your infertility treatment. What are your treatment options? It might be helpful for you to look at some of the processes your physician takes you through and how decisions are made in terms of the treatment opportunities available to you. This will be addressed in the next chapter.

C H A P T E R   3
INFERTILITY TREATMENT OPTIONS

When I was thinking about the content for this book, I gave a lot of thought to what I should say about treatment options. I am not a doctor and did not feel qualified to address the detailed medical aspects of treatment. That information is addressed in other books written by doctors who specialize in infertility treatment. They are the experts. I also struggled with whether or not to include this chapter because the technology is changing so rapidly. Finally, all of us are unique in our infertility treatment needs. Each of us has specific, individual biological, personal, and medical factors that our doctor considers when our case is being reviewed. All of these factors go into the infertility treatment recommendations our doctors make to us.

My husband convinced me, however, that it might be helpful for people reading this book to have a sense of the general types of treatment, and the process and progression commonly involved in your infertility treatment. Hopefully, this will give you an understanding about what to expect, and maybe help you to formulate some questions to raise with your doctor in terms of your own specific treatment needs. I do want to say, though, that everybody's medical situation is different, and you and your doctor are the ones that must make the final determination of the best infertility treatment options for you. This chapter will offer you a general guide about what to consider as you travel through this aspect of your infertility journey.

If after a year of trying to get pregnant you have not had any success, you may want to consider going to a reproductive endocrinologist to decide what the next step should be. Chapter 2 explains the credentials of this type of physician. Your age should also be a consideration in deciding when you consult a reproductive endocrinologist. For example, if you start trying to have a child after the age of thirty-eight, you might want to have a consultation with a reproductive endocrinologist right away. Your chances of having a successful pregnancy beyond that age do get much lower. Consult your internist or gynecologist about whether or not this type of referral would be appropriate for you.

The first time you do meet with an RE you will have a longer appointment. It is helpful to bring your partner to this session as well, if it is possible. Your partner may remember things that you don't. The doctor will ask you both for a lot of information regarding your medical histories. The physician will ask you about your menstrual cycle, how regular it is, and how often it comes. Also, how long does it last? What are your symptoms during your cycle? There will be questions about whether or not either of you have previously tried to have a child, and if you had any successes or failures. Your family history regarding fertility will be explored. Questions will be raised about any current or past medical conditions either of you have had. You will need to share information about what medications you both may be taking. Your habits regarding nutrition, exercise, tobacco, alcohol, and drugs will probably be discussed. Share information regarding any surgeries you may have had in the past and also any allergies you have, especially to medications.

I mentioned in Chapter 2 that having your medical records with you for the meeting will be helpful for you and your doctor. One of the first steps in the process of determining your infertility treatment involves the doctor doing blood tests, getting a urine sample, and possibly performing an ultrasound. There are a multitude of reasons why people have difficulty achieving pregnancy. One of the purposes of the blood tests is to examine the chromosomes of both the man and the woman to detect any abnormalities. The man will probably be asked to give a sperm sample. The doctor is going to use all of this information to look at things like hormone and enzyme levels. The man's sperm count and any abnormalities in the sperm shape or movement will be assessed by your doctor. The woman will probably have a pelvic exam and the doctor will examine your uterus, fallopian tubes, and ovaries. The doctor will look for any evidence of scar tissue in the woman's uterus and fallopian tubes. The woman's protein levels will be measured as well because these impact your ability to ovulate. The doctor will also want to do blood tests and get urine samples from the woman at different times during her cycle to measure hormone levels and protein levels throughout different phases of your menstrual cycle.

One common cause of infertility is pelvic inflammatory disease or PID. PID is a condition where the uterus, ovaries, and fallopian tubes can become inflamed. This is a problem that can be diagnosed and treated. There are medications that can help with PID. In addition to physical diagnoses, your age will have an impact on the treatment recommendations that are made by your doctor. For example, as I said earlier, I was over forty when I began my infertility treatment. My doctor did tests and established a baseline for me, and then had me do a round of ovulation enhancement through medications to see how my body would respond. I reacted poorly to the drug, and had bad side effects and poor hormonal response. After seeing these results and knowing my age, my doctor advised me to skip all other types of infertility treatment and testing because my odds of success were so limited. He recommended I immediately look at an egg donor option. Age is often a big factor in treatment decisions.

In the initial stage of your infertility treatment, you and your partner, in conjunction with your doctor, should have a serious discussion regarding your values and wishes about getting pregnant. Your doctor will give you percentages and statistics related to your likely success rates for getting pregnant. These are based on your age, medical factors, and the type of treatment you will be utilizing. What you and your partner need to weigh in your own hearts and minds is, if a certain procedure has only a ten percent chance of being successful, do you want to try it before you move on to another treatment option? How many times would you try it? Other treatment options might be less desirable, but have a greater possibility of achieving your goal of pregnancy. Do you and your partner feel you need to try every treatment option that would allow you to both be the biological parents, no matter their odds for success, before you would consider other options like using a donor?

These are not easy decisions to make and need to be carefully thought out. Rely on your doctor's expertise to help guide you through this thought process. When you are first beginning your infertility journey, it is really difficult to anticipate and understand the emotional and physical toll infertility treatment can have on you. This experience varies from person to person. Be conscious of these factors as you and your partner make determinations about which direction your infertility treatment should go as you move to different stages. Give yourself permission to change your mind about how long you want to undergo the assorted treatment options available to you. You will gain wisdom and insight during the course of your treatment.

THE COMMON PROGRESSION OF TREATMENTS

Obviously, if your initial examination does reveal that you, your partner, or both of you have a specific medical problem, then this will need to be the early focus of your treatment. Depending on your diagnosis, your doctor may need to address your medical problem surgically. There are some frequent diagnoses that can occur, which may require surgery. Examples of these diagnoses that can impact women include endometriosis, scar tissue in the fallopian tubes, multiple cysts in the ovaries, and fibroids (non-cancerous growths), which are found in the uterus. Examples of potential diagnoses and surgical procedures that would impact men include microsurgical epididymal sperm aspiration and a diagnosis of varicocele, which can be treated surgically. You will find more extensive definitions of these terms in the glossary in Chapter 21.

Let's assume for purposes of discussion that your medical examinations do not turn up any apparent medical problems. Your doctor will ask the woman to keep a daily record of her temperature, or a basal body temperature chart. This will allow your doctor and you to know when you begin to ovulate, and this will help you calculate what your menstrual cycle is. The use of medications is a very common early form of infertility treatment. There are a number of medications that are often used in the early stage of treating women with infertility problems. One common medication used is Clomid or Serophene. This drug helps stimulate ovulation in women. Clomid also helps improve sperm production in men.

Your doctor will also be measuring the woman's follicle stimulating hormone (FSH) and luteinizing hormone (LH) levels. FSH stimulates the follicles that release eggs from the ovaries, and LH is a protein found in the woman's pituitary gland that impacts ovulation. If these levels are not where they should be you will not be able to get pregnant. Pergonal is a frequently used medication to address these problems. It is a mixture of FSH and LH and helps get those levels where they need to be to create effective ovulation and enable you to become pregnant. Urofollitropin is a medicine that is used to stimulate the follicle growth necessary to produce viable eggs. Progesterone is also an important hormone that helps maintain pregnancy in the beginning and must be at a certain level.

Some infertility medications can be taken in pill form. Some of them must be administered by injection. You may be able to inject yourself. I found this to be one of the more difficult aspects of my infertility treatment in spite of the many years I worked in hospitals. I later realized it was the first of a long list of things I would be willing to do in my quest to become a parent. There may be some injections you will not be able to give yourself and your partner will have to assist you with this. This can be a difficult adjustment for both of you. A doctor or nurse can advise you about how to do injections and you should practice on a piece of fruit initially, if you are somewhat queasy about it. This will help desensitize you to this procedure. These injections generally are needed on a daily basis for an extended period of time. Believe it or not, they will eventually become routine for you.

You may experience some side effects from these medications. Always ask your physician about possible side effects. You may feel tired, have headaches, or experience some moodiness. This is not unusual when your hormone levels are stabilizing and your body chemistry is being altered.

There is another test your doctor may want to do to detect other reasons you may not be achieving pregnancy. You may be asked to do a test that is performed quickly after intercourse. It is called a post-coital test (PCT), and its purpose is to determine if the sperm are having trouble moving through the mucus that is found in the cervix. You would be asked to come into your clinic or doctor's office as quickly after intercourse as possible, and then laboratory testing would be done. This test is done around the time of ovulation to determine if there is any incompatibility. Intrauterine insemination is a possible treatment option if your doctor discovers there is some problem with the ability of the sperm to move through cervical mucus. This treatment involves placement of the sperm directly into the cervix or uterine cavity.

ASSISTED REPRODUCTION

Those of us who must look towards in vitro fertilization or assisted reproductive technologies may undergo a number of different treatment regimes. Constant blood tests and urine samples will be an ongoing part of all these infertility treatments. In addition, these regimes involve an assortment of relatively simple surgical procedures that are performed at your fertility clinic. They do not require a general anesthetic. You will need an IV and you will be given a local anesthetic. You may also be given antibiotics to stop any infection. You may be given valium or something else to relax you. But you can be awake for most of these procedures, which generally take less than thirty minutes. For some women, their eggs can have problems attaching to the uterus. Your doctor can place your egg in your uterus. Embryos, which are fertilized eggs, can also be placed in the woman's uterus or fallopian tubes.

You may need to undergo a retrieval, where eggs are removed from the follicles of your ovaries. Drugs are usually administered to enhance ovulation, so that the number of eggs retrieved is higher. The eggs can then be placed in a Petri dish with sperm, in order to be fertilized. The fertilized eggs are developed into embryos, which can later be placed in the woman's uterus or fallopian tubes in a procedure called an embryo transfer. I underwent this procedure. Usually after these procedures you will need to be on bed rest for a day or two to help promote a successful pregnancy. No lifting can be done either. There may be some vaginal bleeding and stomach discomfort. Sperm can also be removed from the man through a relatively simple procedure. Intrauterine insemination involves sperm being placed into the woman's cervix or uterus. Sperm can also be assisted in fertilizing an egg through a micro-manipulation procedure called intracytoplasmic sperm injection (ICSI). These different types of surgeries are being done on a very regular basis today.

Talk with your physician about what type of experience he or she has had doing these procedures and what their success rate is with patients your age. If you do get to the point where you have an embryo or embryos, there are tests that can be done to determine the "quality" of these embryos. Pre-implantation genetic diagnosis is a test where a cell is taken from an embryo and can be tested for any genetic abnormalities. This is done before the embryo is implanted in the woman. Embryos are also physically examined by an embryologist with a microscope. If a problem with the embryo is detected, your doctor will meet with you to discuss the nature of the problem, and determine with you and your partner if implantation of this embryo should proceed.

Most retrievals produce multiple eggs and embryos. In the past, doctors would transfer a higher number of fertilized eggs than they do today. Transferring a high number of fertilized eggs led to high rates of multiple births. Many women were having twins and triplets, and some had even more babies. Carrying multiple fetuses can increase heath risks to the mother and fetuses, and endanger the pregnancy. In some cases, pregnancy reduction is recommended or the prospective parents choose to pursue this alternative. In pregnancy reductions, one or more fetuses are selectively removed, and the others continue to term. Obviously, people have different ethical views about these procedures, and making these decisions can be quite difficult. Pregnancy reductions can also cause a complete miscarriage of the pregnancy. Because of these risks and ethical challenges, transfer practices have been the subject of a lot of research and continue to evolve.

Today, embryology has improved, and embryos are developed longer before being transferred. Currently, embryos are commonly developed to the blastocyst stage before transfer. Fewer of the embryos survive to this stage, but they implant far more frequently in the uterus. The result is that the same odds for achieving a live birth can be achieved with a lower risk of multiple births. In my transfers, only two blastocyst embryos were implanted each time. Once these retrieval and transfer surgeries have been completed and the embryo is in the uterus, your doctor will perform ongoing tests to see if the embryo has properly attached to the uterus and is indeed growing and developing.

The embryos that are not used in the first transfer are frozen, and they can be thawed later for additional transfer attempts. Not all embryos will be viable after being frozen, so often more are thawed than are intended for transfer. Thawed embryos will be carefully

examined by the embryologist, and once again, if there are any problems with an embryo, your doctor will discuss this with you before a
transfer is done. People bring different ethical views to the treatment
of embryos, and you will need to consider your own personal values
around these complex questions. Your doctor and embryologist can
share their professional protocols and help you understand how they
assess the development and viability of your embryos. Fundamentally,
though, you and your partner will have to make the decisions regarding your embryos, including how many to transfer and what should
ultimately happen to any frozen embryos you don't use.

These decisions can be difficult to make, and it is good to
think about them beforehand and know what you want to do. For
example, when you have multiple frozen embryos, you may want to
thaw more than the number you want to transfer to be sure you have
at least that number. You do this to give yourself the best chance to
become pregnant. You might use average viability rates as your guide
for the number of embryos to thaw, and then find that you have more
viable embryos to transfer than you had planned. Now, you can transfer all the viable embryos, but you will increase your risk of multiple
births. In this situation, what would you want to do? The treatment
and assessment of our embryos was an area where we expected more
guidance from our doctor and embryologist. We wanted a clearer
assessment of the embryos than they could give us. They gave us the
odds, and left us to make the decisions. You should know that this is
an area where you and your partner will need to make decisions, and
no one else can really tell you what to do.

When doctors confirm that we are unable to produce our own
healthy eggs or sperm, then we need to decide whether to use a donor.
If you and your partner decide to pursue this option, you will proceed
with assisted reproduction. In the case of egg donation, this is a more
complicated process, because the woman getting the donated eggs
must match her menstrual cycle to that of her donor. Both the donor
and the woman receiving the eggs must be placed on hormone medication to regulate their cycles so they are synchronized. The doctor
will have you and the donor come in for regular blood and urine testing to determine the exact timing of the egg retrieval and embryo
placement in the prospective mother's uterus.

Those of you that decide to use surrogates will face a similar scenario in the sense that the surrogate will have to undergo tests and take medications to prepare her body to be in the proper place in her cycle to have the embryo implanted in her uterus. If the surrogate is to carry your genetic embryo, then you will need to be synchronized for the retrieval, and likewise in the case of an egg donor, if only the father can be a genetic parent. Sometimes, the surrogate will also function as an egg donor, in which case a retrieval is performed, her eggs are fertilized with the father's sperm, and the resulting embryos are transferred to her uterus. Even if your surrogate carries an embryo donated by someone else, she will need to go through the usual assisted reproduction preparation regime. The monitoring process after the implantation is the same as I described above.

THE CHALLENGING JOURNEY

If you are lucky enough to become pregnant, the close monitoring will continue, as your doctor and their staff make sure that you or your baby are having no medical problems. You will continue to receive frequent ultrasounds. Constant blood tests and urine samples will be taken to ensure that your baby is growing and developing normally. This can be a highly stressful time. Around eight weeks into your pregnancy, if everything seems to be all right, your reproductive endocrinologist will graduate you to your obstetrician/gynecologist. This too can be a stressful transition.

When I reflect on my infertility treatment experience and the experiences of others I have talked and worked with, I can't help but recognize that the treatment period of our infertility journey is the most confusing and difficult time. It is a period filled with anxiety, and unexpected roadblocks can occur. It is a time when you feel utterly helpless because so much of what happens is totally out of your control. The outcome of your dream of becoming pregnant is determined by lab tests, blood tests, and surgeries you can't begin to interpret or understand. Your chances of success also depend on the skill level of the professional team entrusted with your future.

There are reasons to be optimistic in terms of the ongoing research being done in the realm of infertility treatment. New procedures are being developed, and established treatment procedures are being honed, all with the ultimate goal of helping you to achieve pregnancy and a healthy baby. Success rate statistics are improving as this body of knowledge grows, and the doctors and support staffs gain experience and expertise. The number of people undergoing infertility treatment continues to grow as well. Don't be afraid to ask questions about the treatment alternatives available to you. Find out about the pros and cons of each of these treatment alternatives in the context of the medical conditions of you and your partner. Remember, the age of the woman is a big factor in the likelihood of success for various treatments. I wish you well on this challenging leg of your infertility journey.

C H A P T E R 4
BALANCING WORK AND INFERTILITY TREATMENT

The media covers lots of stories about the difficulties men and women have balancing family and work. There are many resources available on this topic, but not much information is available on how to balance work and infertility treatment. Thousands of people struggle with this problem on a daily basis. For example: what do you do if you need to leave work to have your blood drawn? This was a real dilemma for me and it caused me quite a bit of stress. Balancing work and infertility treatment was difficult for other people I spoke with too. Here are some stories and ideas about this issue. Hopefully, they will be helpful to you.

There are many questions you can ask when you begin to consider how your infertility treatment will interact with your work. The first question many people want to decide is how transparent to be. Should you tell people at work you are undergoing infertility treatment or keep it private? Thinking about this leads to many other questions. If you decide to tell people, what are you going to say? Will revealing this information impact your job security in any way? What type of job do you have, and how might treatment impact your ability to do your job? What duties in your job description might pose a problem? How far is your place of employment from the place where you will be undergoing your infertility treatment, and how much time will be required going back and forth? With so many questions to consider, it can be daunting to know where to start.

One of the first things you should consider is the type of job you have. This can be critical to deciding how much to reveal about your infertility treatment at work. Women do all kinds of work today, and there are many ways your job can impact your treatment or vice versa. You need to think about a number of issues, including the amount of physical exertion and stress you associate with your job. Stress can be physical or psychological, but both forms can impact your health and potentially your treatment. If you are a professional woman, chances are you put in long hours and deal with a lot of pressures at work. If you are a waitress, cashier, or sales clerk, your job involves hours of standing on your feet. If you are a construction worker, you may be climbing or lifting heavy weights. These types of physical exertion and stress may impact the effectiveness of your infertility treatment. Does your job require a lot of traveling without much notice? This can compromise your infertility treatment (or your job), because you might not be able to miss a lab test or blood draw.

You should spend some time speaking with your doctor about your specific job responsibilities to make sure that they will not have an adverse effect on your infertility treatment. At times, you may have to make a choice between your job and treatment. In certain circumstances, you may need to alter some of your job responsibilities. Maybe there is another job available at your place of employment that offers a better fit with your infertility treatment regime. Unexpected problems can arise during infertility treatment or adoption proceedings. For example, you might be involved in a foreign adoption and face immigration problems that delay your return, or there could be times during you infertility treatment when you must be on bed rest. Can you miss your return date or work at home on these occasions? Do you have the option of going part time or using flextime or taking a leave of absence?

Before you start treatment, you should talk with your doctor about what your treatment needs will likely be and how this is typically scheduled. You need to know what will be required of you in terms of time, tests, meetings, medications, and any others procedures your doctor would do. You should consider how this will mesh with your work schedule, and try to work out a plan in advance. You will need to consider the proximity of where you work to where you will be getting your infertility treatment. For my treatment, I had to have constant blood work and lab work, along with occasional ultrasounds. I made sure there was a clinic near work where I could have this done. Working out a good schedule can be challenging, especially if you decide to keep your infertility treatment private and not tell people at work.

For the most part, I decided not to tell people at work that I was undergoing infertility treatment. Because of this, it was imperative that I had my clinic nearby. I needed to plan to have all of these tests early before work or at my lunchtime. Luckily, I could walk to work from the clinic. It is useful for you to know what medical facilities are near your place of work or travel. In the middle of my treatment I changed jobs, and my new job location made it impossible for me to go to my clinic on a regular basis. I was able to find a satellite office that could offer me the necessary medical procedures and then would forward the information to my clinic. If you do this, make sure the satellite clinic is also covered by your insurance.

As Ann noted in the previous chapter, every medical office has its own culture. When I switched to this new satellite office I quickly realized they were much busier than my other clinic. They booked lots of patients at once and my waiting time was longer. I had to adjust the time I planned away from work to accommodate this new culture. If you know the clinic you are going to is busier, try to book an appointment when you have more time flexibility. I also had to adjust to a new doctor office and support staff after becoming quite comfortable with the staff in my old clinic. It is good to be aware of these types of changes.

WORK, STRESS, AND FERTILITY TREATMENT

While planning for treatment, you should think about any work-related personal pressures or stress issues you face. Stress is often closely linked to work and infertility treatment. I have a personal example. By sheer coincidence the week that I did my first embryo transfer I learned that my office was closing and we were all being "downsized." My office was a great place to work. When I started there, we were a small group of dedicated people, and the company was very successful and grew rapidly. We became a model for the industry and were bought by another, larger company. We thought we would set a new standard inside the larger company, but instead they shut us down. They decided to move our client base to "less expensive" company locations. This decision came out of nowhere. We had no indication that our office was about to close.

It was clearly a very stressful time for me. We had been waiting almost a year for our first retrieval and embryo transfer. I had spent several months taking hormone altering drugs, preparing for the transfer. So much of our future seemed to be riding on those few days. After many months of anticipation, it was all finally happening. I was nervous about my treatment, and whether we would succeed and become parents. I tried to keep living my normal life, going to work and keeping my regular hours, but there was so much at stake in those days of waiting to find out. Then, in the midst of that time, everyone in the office was called down to a meeting. I noticed that our HR person was crying and I knew the news wouldn't be good, and it wasn't—we were all being fired! And not because our business had failed, but because we had done such a great job! We were all shocked, angry, and scared. Now, my stress about the future was compounded. Would I be able to get pregnant and have a baby? Would I need to find another job? After that, I had trouble sleeping and it seemed like I got sick.

My transfer failed and I have always felt there was a connection with my getting the news our office was closing and this failure. It made such a strong impact on me that when we were planning the date for the next embryo transfer I waited until my office had closed down and I was not working. This caused a considerable delay in our next procedure, because I worked until the very last day my office closed. I'm glad I waited, though, because it was hard to see my colleagues leave, and hard to have my last interactions with long-term clients (we were not allowed to tell them what had happened or that we were leaving). I waited so I could minimize any work-related stress as much as possible before my second transfer, and it was successful.

This story illustrates how the stresses of infertility treatment and work can interconnect, and potentially impact, treatment success. I have no way of proving that the office closing negatively impacted my first transfer, but minimizing stress can be important to successful treatment. There is a lot of medical proof that stress can impact hormone levels and affect your immune system. These can both be contributing factors to a successful or unsuccessful pregnancy. Taxed immune systems, as mine was, can even become confused and reject the embryo as though it was a foreign agent in the body. Some doctors even prescribe drugs that suppress the immune system for certain women undergoing particular procedures, and this course of treatment was even offered to me before my second transfer. I decided, however, that my immune reaction was more likely the result of situational stress, which I would be sure to avoid in my next attempted transfer. We clearly all have some type of stress in our work lives, and learning how to deal with this stress is paramount to our overall health. It can also be important to the potential success of our fertility treatment.

If you face particular work-related pressures or stress, you should talk with your doctor about this issue. In addition, your doctor may also be able to alert you to other issues you could face at work. For example, certain medications may cause mood swings, or they may have other side effects that impact your work. It may be difficult for you to concentrate, read, or focus because of medications you are taking. You may need to miss work because of surgical procedures, or it might be advisable to take some extra time away from the stress of work for recuperation. You should discuss all these potential issues with your doctor as you plan for the beginning of your treatment.

THE PRIVACY QUESTION

Once you know the parameters of your treatment and have done a little planning, you will be better able to answer the question of how transparent to be. You will need to consider who to tell at work, and what and when to tell them about your infertility treatment. The people I've talked with gave me a complete range of answers on what to tell co-workers and how open to be. Someone in my office shared every intimate detail of her infertility treatment with all of us. There are others I know who have chosen not to tell anybody. In some instances you may need to share this information with your immediate supervisor or boss. Unexpected things do occur, and you may need to have some flexibility at work. At times, it's good to have a confidante, too. Think about what will make you feel most comfortable. Think about the climate and culture in your workplace and consider what feels right for you. You want to create a situation where you have as much support as possible without feeling people are being intrusive and without fear of losing your job.

My own experience around transparency was mixed. I had two jobs during the course of my infertility treatment. In my first job there were a couple of people at the office who I told about my infertility treatment. At my second job, I kept my treatment quiet for the most part. I was working when the call came that my initial embryo transfer attempt had failed and I was not pregnant. What a tough week that was! It felt good to have some people at work I could trust and who were close by. It was comforting to be able to talk with somebody immediately, when I needed to. They were very supportive. This was a time when I had to find the strength to continue and complete my workday, while coping with so much difficult news.

On the other hand, at my second job, I initially chose to keep my infertility treatment private. I had my second embryo transfer in the two week period between jobs, so I would be totally free of work and could relax. Though I got pregnant, I wasn't sure what the outcome would be yet, or how this might affect my position at the office. I was also concerned that people (with the best of intentions) might ask me questions about my treatment that I didn't feel comfortable answering. I decided if things did not go well this might be difficult for me to handle. When I suffered my miscarriage after my wedding, there were many people who had known I was pregnant, but never heard about the miscarriage. They would innocently ask me questions about my pregnancy, and I would have to tell them that it had ended and relive that sorrow again. They always had the best intentions and were always very sorry. Sometimes, it's easier to deal with the ups and downs of infertility by keeping it mostly private, and sharing the information with only a close circle of people.

There is another story I recall from the period when I was unsuccessful with my infertility treatment. During that time, one colleague adopted a child and another had a baby. There were office parties celebrating these occasions. It was a bit uncomfortable for me to participate in these parties, but I consciously chose to stay, partly because I hadn't told many people about my treatment and leaving would have seemed strange. Sometimes it's difficult to be in the position of helping people celebrate their new parenting in the midst of infertility treatment. If you know a party like this is going to take place, you can choose not to attend. If you have disclosed your infertility treatment to a supervisor, you can request that you be allowed to leave the office and make up the work another time. You might also let your colleagues know that you wish them well. You can share with them your current infertility struggle, but you shouldn't feel that you have to explain your feelings. It can be very difficult to be around people celebrating their new parenthood, and sometimes the challenges of this are compounded by privacy concerns.

Keeping your treatment private at work can be challenging. You should think about whether there is a private space available to you at your workplace. When your doctor or nurse calls you with information, is there a place where you can go while you are on the telephone? You may want to discuss when and where your doctor or their staff will contact you with pertinent information regarding your treatment. This can be important to maintaining the level of privacy you feel is appropriate at work. What if you need some time alone to cope with news or elements of your treatment? Is there a room or office you can use when you need it?

In my case, there was nowhere private for me to make or receive personal calls, so I had to go outside my office floor to contact my nurse or my doctor with questions. I remember the day I found out I was pregnant with my daughter, Grace. I had to walk outside and across the street to collect myself and calm down enough to return to work, so I could function the way I needed to. This ongoing juggling act at work can certainly create additional stress for you, which is yet another reason you want to work with a compassionate doctor and nurse.

As my pregnancy continued, I really struggled with the question of how transparent to be at my second job. I had worked previously with the person who offered me the job, and my new boss knew that I would be a competent, hard worker. I was very grateful to her for giving me this career opportunity. At the same time I was committed to continuing my infertility treatment. Given my age and the kind of infertility treatment I was having, I had a real sense that time was running out for me. I also had no guarantees that my infertility treatment would be successful. I did not want to do anything to jeopardize my new job. I felt very badly about not being totally honest with my new boss. Frankly, I was in a new work culture and I was not sure how the news of my pregnancy or infertility treatment would be received. This was another source of stress for me. I wasn't sure how much I should tell my employer.

I ultimately chose to share information about my treatment with my human resources representative, who was invaluable in helping me navigate some of my insurance issues. I knew I could trust her to respect my confidentiality. She also was extremely helpful in putting me in touch with people who could clarify specifics about my insurance coverage for infertility related treatment.

One of my interviewees, Kate, provides a flip-side example of transparency. Kate is an attorney and she decided to openly share her plan to do an international adoption. She told me that her co-workers and boss were incredibly supportive. They gave her the flexibility she needed to be away for weeks when she went to China to get her daughter. She spent time discussing her cases with colleagues before she left, so all her cases were well-covered. Kate knew she planned to return to her job after the adoption, but she also planned to take a leave from work under the Family Medical Leave Act. This law allows you to take time from work to care for a family member, and many people make use of this act when new babies are born.

The Family Medical Leave Act was instated so people could take care of family members when necessary, without fear of losing their jobs. The act protects your employment, but does not guarantee you the same job and does not apply to all employers. You can ask your supervisor or human resources staff about the Family Medical Leave Act and how it applies to you. You should get the specifics regarding how a leave like this would affect your salary, benefits, and return to your current job. It's not enough to know what the law says. Different employers have different approaches to family leave, with some being quite supportive and progressive, while others view it very negatively. In some workplaces, family leave is viewed as a disruption of the work environment, and some employers take a more "punitive" approach to compliance. The job waiting for you when you come back may not be the job you had or one you want.

The culture in some workplaces is still pretty archaic and non-supportive. You may want to be transparent about your infertility treatment generally, but decide that it would be better not to tell people at work because of the situation there. You may wonder if revealing this information will impact your job security, and in some situations it could. If there appears to be a real possibility of putting your job in jeopardy, you can consult an attorney to discuss your legal rights. In some situations, knowing what to say can be a legal matter, but fertility treatment or pregnancy should not be grounds for putting your job in jeopardy. You do have legal recourse in these situations, and you are under no obligation to reveal your treatment to an employer.

WORKING WOMEN AND MOTHERHOOD

The outcome of fertility treatment is never certain, yet in many employment settings there can be an assumption that, if you are undergoing treatment, you may want to leave employment and have a family. This connects with a lot of societal expectations that have been linked to the lives of women and work for generations. My husband has an aunt in her nineties who has a favorite story she likes to tell. When she first got married she was working as a bank teller. The bank had a rule that it would not employ any woman that was married. This policy was based on more than the Victorian "propriety" of those old days. The bank made the calculated assumption that married women would have babies and then leave their jobs. My husband's aunt and uncle were both very young when they first met, and they eloped without announcements or fanfare. She was afraid of losing her job, because they needed her income to afford their apartment. She would take off her wedding ring on the way to work. One day she was riding the streetcar home and she put her wedding ring back on. A co-worker from the bank saw her wearing the ring and revealed her secret. Her boss confronted her the next day and asked the aunt if she was married. She confessed her secret and lost her job.

While today's social conventions have changed, a pregnancy stigma remains in many professions and workplaces. Obviously, you can be married and work today, but being pregnant can cause challenges in the workplace. This is particularly true as the culture of work expands and more women move into traditional "men's jobs." A pregnant construction worker, for example, might have to file for disability. Beyond the potential physical challenges of being pregnant on the job, employers face the same age-old question asked by the bank: will our pregnant employees keep working, or will we incur a lot of expense during their pregnancies and then need to replace them? This question lies at the root of the pregnancy stigma today; just at it did several generations ago.

As professional women work their way up, they can still encounter a "glass ceiling" in many workplaces. Sometimes subtle limitations on their advancement are triggered or reinforced when professional women decide to pursue motherhood. For many professional women, motherhood is put off to pursue their career. Women who are fast risers with high potential can find their advancement slowed and career options limited once they decide to have kids. For many women this happens in the prime of their careers, when they are still young and have real opportunities for advancement. Unfortunately, according to their biological clock, they are "getting old" to become pregnant. This can seem to create hard choices.

The percentage of women in high-ranking business and political positions in this country is climbing, but it is still relatively low. It appears that, even today, women are often put in the position of having to choose between devoting themselves to their careers or their families. Sometimes, it is society that creates this tension (often through pressures of the workplace), but more frequently it is a tension within us that we feel ourselves. It seems whatever choice we make, there can be an element of guilt or dissatisfaction associated with our inability to simultaneously do our job and be a good mother. It's hard to strike a balance and pursue either at the level you would like. This balancing act is far more frequently placed on women than men, and in the work world there can be a preconception that when women become mothers they may be less professionally oriented.

Sue, one of my interviewees, was a professional woman. Her job was not a daily 9-5 type of position. Her hours varied, depending on the needs of the client, and she worked as a consultant. This gave her flexibility to schedule her treatment as needed without necessarily telling anyone. Treatment was one thing, but having a baby would be different. She had decided that if she was successful at having a child she wanted to be a full-time, stay-at-home mother. She had decided she would leave her job when the time came and she was having a baby.

Being in treatment is no guarantee that you will succeed and have children, so sometimes the solution to the issue of professional transparency is to wait, like Sue did. However, like Sue, you should also think about whether or not you plan on returning to work if you do become a parent. That was one of the first questions my supervisor asked me when I told her I was pregnant.

I waited until I was done with my first trimester before I shared my pregnancy news with my boss. My doctor told me that was the time of highest risk for the pregnancy. Once I conquered that hurdle, I felt more optimistic about my pregnancy going to term, and I wanted my supervisor to know I was pregnant as soon as possible. My response to her question about whether I would return to work was that I planned to come back. Once my daughter was born, however, I knew in my heart that I wanted to be with her on a full-time basis. Luckily, our financial situation allowed me this flexibility. Not all women who would like to make this choice are able to do it.

I did tell my boss quickly when I decided to leave my job and be a full time mother, and she was very gracious about it. It was really a conversation I was dreading, but she made it easy for me. If you are ambivalent about what you will do after you are a parent, you may want to share these feelings with your employer, if you feel comfortable doing it. Chances are, your employer and co-workers will be wondering what you intend to do, and shared clarity may be good in the workplace, no matter what your intentions. It's not always possible to decide in advance what you will do. In this case, you may be able to negotiate a timeframe with your boss, and set a date for making the ultimate determination about continuing your job or remaining at home on a full-time basis. Often, it's best to make this decision after you become a parent.

This decision is subject to all kinds of societal pressures. Many people feel that parenthood changes their lives completely. It is common for people to feel they will need to move to a bigger living space or a better neighborhood. Along with this, comes the need for more money, not less. The financial pressure to keep working can increase when you have children, and this can be at odds with the desire to stay home. Not all women want to stay home, or should they. In many households the woman makes more money than the man does.

I believe it is useful for women and men to spend some time thinking about the balance of life at work and life at home. As a woman, you should consider how your maternity would impact your view of your work-self. We don't really focus on that much when we are in the midst of infertility treatment. Is a lot of your self-esteem tied up with the work that you do? Giving that up, even to be a mother, may have a negative impact on how you look at yourself. If you tend to be a high-achieving, competitive person in your work environment, then giving that up may be the wrong decision for you. The world of motherhood is an entirely different, unfamiliar realm, one more difficult to control and direct. It is a huge adjustment. I will look at these issues more in Chapter 14, Parenting After Infertility.

WORK AND INFERTILITY

Infertility treatment can last a long time. Because success is unpredictable, most women who are working keep working, and it's probably good to try and maintain your normal life as much as possible during treatment. Sometimes, making life changes in anticipation of treatment only raises the pressure and stress of the inevitable waiting. If you don't get pregnant in early attempts, the sense of urgency can be compounded. It's best to approach infertility treatment with patience and hope, knowing that success can take time. For most working women, this means staying on the job.

If you are faced with this situation, you need to determine what level of transparency is appropriate in your workplace for you. If you prefer privacy, you should consider how comfortable you would be with keeping information about your infertility treatment a secret. Think about the relationship you have with your employer and the culture of work at your place of employment. Will your infertility treatment hinder your ability to function on the job in any way? Will disclosing your situation result in any negative consequences? Is there anybody else at work that has been in this situation? If you can, talk to somebody with experience and find out what choices they made regarding transparency and infertility treatment and what the outcome was.

If you do choose to disclose, you need to sort out how and what you will tell your employer regarding your infertility treatment. You should have a clear understanding of how much detail to go into and what you will say about your treatment's time demands. I would suggest you be prepared to emphasize all of the things you are doing to make sure your infertility treatment is not interfering with your work. If your treatment is time-ended, then give this information to your employer so it can be addressed appropriately. Maybe there is somebody at work who can cover for you when you need to miss work. If you can negotiate that type of arrangement with a co-worker, then discuss this with your employer.

There are many ways to be pro-active about meshing your treatment and your job. You can try having lab work and blood tests done before or after work. If you have to miss work and can make it up another time, then offer to negotiate about this with your employer. If you have a job that is seasonal, perhaps you can arrange with your doctor to have more intensive treatment done during the off-season. If you anticipate you may need time off of work, you should consider being proactive and discussing this with your employer. For example, if you will need bed rest after a surgical procedure, you can let your boss know when you anticipate this will happen, and that it will only be for a day or so. Even without going into many details, you can let your boss know that you will be undergoing a medical procedure, and that the duration of your time off is based on your doctor's recommendations. If adoption is the direction you are going, you could discover that you need to be away for three weeks for an international adoption. For a domestic adoption you literally may have only one day's notice that the time of the adoption has arrived. You may want to discuss the parameters of these time demands with your supervisor.

Whether or not you choose to reveal your infertility situation, you can always be in control of the information. The level of privacy you maintain is up to you, but however private you choose to be, you will still need to manage your communication. Thinking about what to say in advance is usually quite helpful, and being proactive about communication is usually a good idea. Have a plan about your treatment, and know what you are going to say about this before the conversation begins. Remember, you can choose to discuss your infertility treatment with your boss, supervisor, or human resources representative, and then ask them to respect your confidentiality. You can explain the nature of your treatment or adoption plans in as little or as much detail as you want. You can nothing or you can simply say you have wanted a child, and now you are now working with a doctor, or adoption agency, to help make this dream become a reality.

The juggling of work and infertility treatment requires lots of time and soul searching. It is a delicate balance that reminds me of a circus performer doing the high wire act. Being proactive in terms of planning what you will disclose to people in your work world and how you will disclose it will require time and careful thought. You should attempt to take control of some of these difficult aspects of your infertility journey in advance. Discuss how to do this with you partner and maybe some close friends who can give you an objective perspective. You will need to weigh the pros and cons of guarding your privacy vs. risking problems at your job. Try to determine, as best you can, what will be the least stressful option for you.

To prepare yourself, you will need to think carefully about the nature of the work you do and the type of demands it makes on you mentally, emotionally, and physically. Carefully consider the culture of your office and the personalities and relationships you share with your colleagues, supervisors, and human resources staff (when they are available). Speak with your doctor and support staff or your adoption personnel about the frequency and nature of the time demands that will be made on you during the infertility treatment or adoption proceedings. You should also think ahead, and consider what you would do, if you were successful in becoming a parent. Would you want to keep working full-time, take a leave, reduce hours or stay home? Don't feel like you have to make decisions in advance and then always stick to them. Whatever you think you want to do now may change later, and that's okay. But be prepared and thinking in advance about what and how to communicate. Stress management, introspection, and thoughtful planning can make all the difference in this part of your infertility journey.

CHAPTER 5
HEALTH INSURANCE
AND PAYING FOR TREATMENT

We are all painfully aware that the costs of healthcare are continuing to skyrocket. Regardless of the type of infertility treatment you are undergoing, it is safe to say that there will be high costs associated with your treatment. In both my personal and professional experience, I learned that you need to spend time understanding your insurance long before you get your first claim. In fact, you should spend some time going over your insurance options, and be sure to pick the right plan before you begin treatment. In this chapter I will offer you information on the questions to ask, the factors to weigh, and the specific components to look for when determining what choices to make regarding your insurance coverage. I will also share with you some of the strange ways that the healthcare system "works" around insurance and money.

Insurance coverage is a huge issue for all of us when we have healthcare needs. Infertility treatment in particular has numerous costs, no matter which type of treatment you are utilizing. There are costs associated with seeing your doctor or nurse, buying your medications, and having your blood and laboratory work done. Not all health insurance policies will cover infertility treatment, or some may limit the types of treatment covered. You should also keep in mind that if you use a donor or surrogate, your costs may more than double. You are responsible for paying for their treatment, and they will not be covered by your health insurance. Fertility clinics, like many "elective" healthcare providers, tend to charge high prices for services that are often not covered by insurance.

It is very important for your doctor and the office support staff to be skilled at dealing with the insurance companies. This requires knowledge, patience, and being proactive. The way they document and submit your medical information can make a big difference in what gets covered by your insurance company. Fostering a good relationship with someone in your clinic or practice can help assure that there is good communication around issues of insurance coverage. As the patient, you are in the best position to be proactive about pursuing insurance claims, but your medical team can also help. You will need to keep good records and understand the basic "system" of healthcare finance. In this chapter, I will try to help you understand how to deal with your insurance company and medical provider, and what to do if your insurance policy does not initially appear to cover your infertility treatment. I will also look into what options you have when your insurance does not cover an infertility treatment you need. There can be a lot of money at stake, and yet many people don't follow up because the whole system is too confusing.

My husband and I had three different insurance companies during the course of my treatment. All of them had different types of coverage. It was terribly frustrating for me, trying to determine which doctor's tests, medications, and treatments were covered under each insurance plan. It's often not easy to make sense out of your coverage, and it is important to know what questions you should ask. There are three possible scenarios for your healthcare coverage. You can have complete coverage, partial coverage, or no coverage. If you get health care through work, you will likely have the option of enrolling in several different plans. You need to know what choices are available to you, and what coverage makes the most sense in your given treatment situation.

You might think that complete coverage is always the most desirable, but this is not necessarily the case. Complete coverage is provided by health maintenance organizations (HMOs). If you are in an HMO plan, you must use their doctors, go through their referral system, and have all your treatment done through the HMO facilities. Generally speaking, when you do this your coverage should be close to 100%. I would encourage you to consult your individual HMO plan to insure this is the case. You need to be sure that fertility treatment is covered by your HMO plan and that the clinics and doctors in your HMO are the right ones for your treatment. HMOs will sometimes limit your choices of treatment, and the best fertility clinics may not be in your HMO.

Most other insurance plans are written with partial coverage in mind. You will pay premiums in exchange for partial coverage, and generally the more you pay in premiums the better your coverage will be. But you have to understand how insurance works and choose your policy carefully, particularly with regard to fertility coverage. Not all insurance policies cover fertility treatment, or the procedures covered may be limited. It is important to know exactly what is covered when you are assessing a particular policy. Even then, figuring out the trade-offs in cost and coverage can be quite complicated.

Most insurance policies eventually provide 100% coverage. But you usually have to pay a certain dollar amount "out of pocket" before your coverage becomes 100%. Your out-of-pocket is the money you pay directly to your provider, and usually this amount has a limit or cap. When you reach your policy's out-of-pocket limit, you stop paying and your insurance pays 100%. The combination of your out-of-pocket limit and your annual insurance premiums represents your total potential healthcare costs in a single year. Your out-of-pocket limit is reached by paying deductibles and co-pays.

The first money paid is always your deductible. Deductibles can range from one hundred to several thousand dollars. You must pay this amount of money to your medical providers before your insurance coverage is triggered, and the insurance company begins to contribute payment to your medical costs. Afterwards, you and your insurance company split the costs, and your portion of this is your "co-pay." Your co-pay portion is calculated as a percentage of your healthcare costs. This percentage is set in your policy and is usually around 20-40% of the costs, with the insurance company paying the remaining 60-80% of the costs. Sometimes your co-pay percentage will vary for different areas of coverage, and you will pay higher or lower percentages for doctor visits, hospital stays, surgery, drugs, etc. You continue to pay your co-pay amounts until you reach your policy's out-of-pocket limit, at which point 100% coverage kicks in (up to the limit of your policy's coverage).

Effectively balancing the trade-offs of cost and coverage can be challenging. Choosing a deductible, for example, can be very confusing. Having lower deductibles means you have more coverage (your insurance kicks in sooner), but you will also have higher premiums.

Many people prefer to have higher deductibles because this helps to reduce the cost of premiums. You will need to take a close look at the numbers to really understand this trade-off. Often, higher deductibles and co-pays end up being cheaper because you are assuming more of the initial risk. But this difference can be washed out if you reach your out-of-pocket limit, as can happen when you are pursuing expensive fertility treatments. Having a good, advance estimate of your annual treatment costs can help you sort out which combination of premiums, deductibles, co-pays, and out-of-pocket limits makes the most sense for you. You should use your assumed treatment costs to compare different policies and their coverage and costs.

CHOSING YOUR INSURANCE POLICY

Selecting an insurance policy is a difficult task at best. Deciphering the language can be intimidating and frustrating. Also, at the time you selected your insurance, you may not have been aware that you would need coverage for infertility treatment. Once you know you need infertility treatment, the best place to start is to review your insurance booklet very carefully. See what it says and how coverage applies to the type of treatment you will need. Keep in mind that the insurance company may use very vague language, and try not to highlight areas of treatment that are not covered.

You will need to carefully explore what differences there are for you between health insurance plans. You should compare policies in relation to monthly costs, deductibles, out-of-pocket expenses, and the percentage of coverage you get. In relation to infertility treatment there will be medication costs, laboratory costs, possibly surgical expenses, and ultrasounds. Look closely at the insurance plan you are considering and see what the coverage is in all these areas, particularly your coverage for drugs and elective surgical procedures. You should also see if there is coverage for inpatient hospitalization, in case you need to be in the hospital overnight for a procedure.

If the insurance booklet does not address an area you are trying to compare, you do have options. If you work for a company that has a human resources department, contact that department and see if they have any additional materials from the insurance company that describe the benefit package. You can also ask specifically for materials regarding infertility treatment, or if you have disclosure issues at work, you can contact the insurance company directly. Ask for additional information and materials about your benefit package, and be specific with your questions if you can be. Sometimes, all the insurance company sends you is a "bare bones" description of your coverage.

If you work for a large company, they generally have sessions one or two times a year where they do an open enrollment, which is your chance to opt for a particular insurance benefit plan. Educate yourself about the different types of insurance that your company has to offer you. There may be significant differences for example between a managed care, or HMO, plan and other non-HMO benefit plans. In my case when we switched to an HMO plan we received 100% coverage. This wasn't luck. It was a conscious choice I made, based on research about my insurance options and whether the HMO would cover my treatment.

When applying for insurance you must be totally honest about your medical history. If you are not, you risk losing coverage. All insurance companies look at pre-existing conditions. If you are not honest and they learn about a pre-existing condition, they have the right to deny your coverage. If you have had previous infertility treatment, you will need to disclose this. If you think you might want to change insurance plans, it's always a good idea to make the change before you start treatment.

There are many types of insurance programs to choose from. You obviously need to look at the entire plan, not just infertility coverage, as you assess the kinds of healthcare needs you have. For example, you may be on costly medications or there may be types of treatment you need on a regular basis. Think about these issues and whether you have regular annual checkups that include special tests, such as mammograms. Here are some specific initial questions that are important to ask when you are selecting the coverage that is right for you. Be sure to get clear answers from the insurance company or your employer, and remember to document their responses:

- What is the deductible for your plan?
- Ask for a list of hospitals and doctors that are covered in the plan, and find out if your doctor and hospital are on their list. Some people choose plans based on whether their chosen doctor or hospital participates. How important is this to you?
- Are there any co-pays for medical treatment such as doctor visits or for medications?
- What is the coverage for prescription drugs? Are there restrictions on where these medications can be purchased? Many programs have a mail-in medication service that may be more cost effective for you. Ask about this.
- What is the out-of-pocket maximum for you? Ask about this in terms of individual out-of-pocket and family out-of-pocket expenses.
- What are the differences between in-network and out-of-network costs for you? In-network providers are selected by the insurance company to be preferred providers under your plan. Do you have the option of seeing out-of-network providers and still retaining some coverage? How much more would this cost?
- Where can you get specific written information regarding this plan and its providers? Be sure you have this information about providers before you make a selection.
- If you are not happy with your doctor, clinic, or hospital what are your options under the plan?
- How are insurance claims handled under the plan? For example, HMO programs often file the claims for you. How important is it for you to have somebody else handle this piece of it? Remember that when you select an HMO, they may be the ones to decide which doctors you see, and when. So think about the specific healthcare priorities that you and your family have.
- If you are not happy with the plan you select, when will be the next opportunity to make a change and what is the process?
- What options do you have to appeal a decision? What is the time limit for making an appeal? Who do you need to contact? What is the time frame for a final determination? What information is needed to make an appeal?

Of course, you should be sure to spend some time looking specifically at the coverage for infertility treatment, too. RESOLVE does put out written information regarding insurance, and I would recommend you contact your local office or the national office in Somerville, Massachusetts to request this information. You can find out how to contact RESOLVE in Chapter 22. RESOLVE has a nominal fee to purchase this information. The following questions about infertility treatment were included in the handout I got from their "Questions to Ask" series:

- How long do you have to try to become pregnant before being referred for infertility tests/treatment?
- What required testing must be completed before you are referred to an infertility specialist?
- If infertility was diagnosed before signing up with the plan (pre-existing condition), will the plan pay for care related to infertility?
- Does the plan require or allow you to seek a second opinion? Will it pay for that visit?
- Is there a maximum payment cap on infertility treatment coverage or on specific treatments?
- Does the plan cover the costs for experimental therapies and will it explain what is experimental?
- Is infertility treatment paid for when you are away from home (e.g. ultrasound and lab work while traveling)?(10)

These are some of the questions from the RESOLVE list. Remember to get detailed information about the kind of infertility treatment you will be doing. You should also be aware of other potential treatments you may need in the future, and try to get coverage information about these, too. For example, if you know you are going to have egg donor treatment, you would want to know whether the insurance covers the costs of freezing and maintaining the embryos. You should know whether there are any specific restrictions regarding treatment in or out of state. You can ask if there is a limit to the number of retrievals that are covered. If you are working with a surrogate, you should find out what treatment costs will be covered for the surrogate mother. Be sure to ask about your coverage for medications and any restrictions that may apply. You should also examine questions about surgery coverage closely for both men and women. Remember that forty percent of infertility problems are male related, which can often result in surgery, too.

It is a given that you will probably need to take some kind of medication, when you undergo infertility treatment. Know this up front and ask for the specifics about your drug coverage in advance. Your doctor should be able to list the different medications they may prescribe in your case. You can check this list against the drug coverage in your insurance policy. It is important to note that there may be specific medications that are covered, but only in particular quantities or doses, and things like syringes may or may not be covered. Some insurance programs cover oral medications but not fertility medications that require injection, so be sure to find out about this. Ask both your doctor and the insurance company about the different forms of medications you might take (including generics), so you don't find out later that your doctor recommends one for your specific, ongoing treatment, but your insurance company will only pay for the other. Drugs are an ever-increasing portion of healthcare costs today.

CAUTIONARY TALES OF INSURANCE

Even if you take the time to figure out your coverage and costs at the beginning, you aren't done dealing with the challenges of insurance. For example, we had our costs all figured out, and then my employer switched insurance providers in the middle of the year. As a result, we "lost" the out-of-pocket we had already accumulated in that partial year, and had to start over with a new deductible and zero out-of-pocket. After looking at the insurance options open to you, you might decide to change plans in order to improve coverage. But you should consider the impact this could have on any out-of-pocket you have already accumulated. It might look like you have more coverage, but the combination of having two policies in a single year could end up costing you more.

Deductibles and out-of-pocket limits can also be tricky. You should always make sure you have a good understanding about whether your policy's deductibles are per person or per family. Often, each covered individual has their own deductibles to fulfill. Also be sure to find out if your insurance plan has a maximum out-of-pocket amount for you, and whether this is per person or per family and how these apply. Some policies have great coverage at lower costs, but no out-of-pocket limit! With this kind of policy, 100% coverage never kicks in, no matter how high your medical bills go.

You will also need a clear understanding of what services are included in your coverage. Coverage can vary within a given policy, and so, for example, you might find that routine medical visits have great coverage, but surgical procedures do not. Often, it is equally important to know what services are excluded under your insurance plan. If a medical service is excluded you will be responsible for the entire cost. The insurance benefits booklets are not always very specific about these exclusions. This can be particularly true with regard to infertility treatments, so focus on the areas of treatment that are pertinent to you, and be sure to get clarification. You should talk directly with an insurance claims representative and your human resources department. Be sure you get a consistent response, and not just one person's "interpretation," and remember, the best way to know you have the right answer is to get it in writing. It's always preferable to have responses in writing to these kinds of questions.

If you are in a PPO plan, or preferred provider plan, you are not necessarily required to work with healthcare providers that are in your healthcare network. But, if you see somebody outside of this network, your costs will likely be substantially higher. With infertility treatment you may be referred to several different doctors or specialists, and you cannot assume that one PPO doctor will refer you to another in-network provider. You should always confirm with your insurance company that the providers you are being referred to are indeed in your PPO plan. This can save you lots of money. These are a few of the hard lessons you learn from dealing with insurance companies, and hopefully you can benefit from this information before you have to deal with this experience yourself. Here are some of the insurance lessons learned by the people I interviewed.

Eliza and Todd had problems with their insurance covering the cost for the intrauterine insemination treatments she needed. They knew the treatment would be expensive. Todd had the option with his company of open enrollment, when he could switch from one insurance plan to another during the year. Many companies offer this option once or twice a year, but some employers do not allow you to change your insurance at all. Todd and Eliza chose to switch their insurance coverage. He explored the coverage in a different insurance plan offered by his company, keeping in mind what types of infertility treatment his doctor anticipated they might need. He selected the plan that offered the most coverage for their designated infertility treatment. Todd said: "I knew that having insurance coverage was a rarity—that my one insurance company picked up any of it. We spent $80,000 out of our pocket."

Switching insurance policies to get some coverage doesn't always minimize your out-of-pocket expense. Even with insurance coverage, fertility treatment can be very expensive, particularly when treatment stretches out over long periods of time, as it did for Todd and Eliza. When treatment goes on for years, your annual out-of-pocket limit has to be reached each year. In addition, switching insurance can also trigger issues around pre-existing conditions. If you have had infertility treatment in the past, when you try to start up with a new insurance company, they may claim your infertility is a pre-existing condition and attempt to exclude it from coverage. You should know what your options are, including if and when you can alter your insurance coverage and what effect switching will have. Know before you switch if the insurance company intends to exclude anything from your policy.

Sue and Howard provide another example of real life experience. They live in the state of Illinois, where, thanks to the hard work of a group of dedicated women, state law mandates insurance coverage in certain instances. The Illinois Family Building Act applies to any company that has twenty-five or more employees, is headquartered in Illinois, and is not self-insured. The company must have a traditional health plan through a third party insurer, and the insurance policy must be issued inside the state of Illinois. If these conditions are met, the law requires that the company's insurance plan cover four cycles of advanced reproductive technology in your lifetime.

You might think this kind of law would always be a good thing, but insurance companies can respond to legislation in unusual ways. This law directly impacted Sue and Howard, but not necessarily the way it was intended to. "I had gone to some seminars," Howard said, "and was told you need to be in a group plan to get covered." Howard had been told that their Blue Cross coverage was under a group plan, but this proved to be wrong. "I called Blue Cross and one person would say it was covered," Howard said, "and another person would say it wasn't. It turns out the policy I got was not a group policy. It was an individual policy and that delayed stuff for a year." He advises others: "Make sure the person you are talking to is answering the right question."

That was not the end of Howard and Sue's story, though. "We went through four cycles of insemination," Sue said, "and we were told we had to do it for insurance purposes." They would not have undergone all these treatments, which had a very low probability of success, but they needed to have medical documentation in order to get coverage for the next step in their infertility journey. Eventually, Sue and Howard's outcome was a positive one and they ended up with good coverage. "I got on my work policy, a group policy, and we had 80% coverage," Howard said. "We had a $2000 maximum deductible and then they paid 100% after that." It wasn't easy for them to get good coverage. It required patience, knowledge, and a willingness to deal with artificial hurdles created by the insurance company in response to the law.

DEALING WITH YOUR PROVIDERS

Whether it's your doctor or your insurance company, dealing with providers can be very challenging. Howard described a typical frustrating experience he and Sue had regarding their medication coverage. "I had to fight to get money back for the drugs," he said, "anything I prepaid for. One of the drugs we got in a small package of dosage and a large package of dosage and I had prepaid. For some reason, I got both in a couple of days. Sure enough, the insurance paid for the small one, which was like $300, but they wouldn't pay for the large one, which was like $1500. It took me two years of telling them, 'Look you paid for this drug here but not this one—same drug but different vials.' It turns out anything over $600 they had to review. I would talk to someone and they would say fax it in; I would fax in five pages and never send them the original copy. I would call back two months later and they would say, 'Oh, we don't have any records of this.' Then I would have to start all over. It took me two years. There were a couple of $1500 checks I finally got."

Sue said that handling the insurance was one of the most supportive things Howard did for her during their infertility journey. She explained: "I did the paperwork for the first two years, and there was a point when Howard took it over. And that felt huge for me. I felt so lightened up. Hearing him say, 'I am now going to do this.' I didn't have to worry about it anymore."

In our case, I had more experience than my husband did with insurance, so I did the paperwork. It is incredibly important to keep a workable file that you can use because the amount of insurance paperwork you will collect is enormous. You will be getting correspondence from your insurance company that is an Explanation of Benefits, or an EOB. This is not a bill. It is a form that will show you the date of your service, the service provider, your account number, and what type of service you are being billed for. There are categories that show you what the total billed amount is, as well as what payment is allowed. The EOB will show you what your savings are, what is being applied to the deductible, what the insurance payment is, and what your out-of-pocket portion of the payment is. Each EOB contains very important information and you should save all of these forms.

One of the first lessons in medical billing is that the initial amount charged on the bill you get from a doctor or hospital is almost always wrong. This is an infuriating and frustrating aspect of health-care billing. If you have insurance, then there is likely a negotiated rate between your provider and your insurance company for particular services. The first bill you receive from a doctor or hospital almost never reflects the negotiated rate. Instead it shows the "retail" cost of your medical service, as though you walked in without insurance and had no negotiated discount. In insurance language, these eventual cost reductions reflect "reasonable and customary costs," but each agreed upon fee is negotiated between an individual healthcare provider and insurance company. In reality, there is no "customary" fee for a service, but negotiated fees are always less than the standard billing fee. The bottom line is: never pay a medical bill until you see the EOB.

You need to cross reference all of your EOBs with the corresponding bills you get. You can match them up by their date of service and provider. The dollars billed should match. Make a note about what has been paid by insurance and what has not. Write down what you paid and when, and the check number or method of payment. Save credit card slips when you get them back. You should only have to pay the amount that the EOB says. You should not pay any bill until you have an EOB. This is the only way to confirm that the bill was properly submitted to your insurance company. Attach the bills to the matching EOB, and file them in a way that you can easily access them. I keep mine filed by date of service. I realize that this sounds like a lot of work, but the payoff is that it can save you a lot of money.

Let me give you an example of just what can happen. I recently got a medical bill for over $600. I realized that I had never gotten an EOB, and when I called the provider, I learned they had sent my bills to the wrong place. As a result of my call, they properly readjusted my claim. I ultimately paid $60 on that bill and my insurance company paid the rest of the claim. There are also times when double-billing can occur, where you are billed for the same service more than once. This is another good reason to save your records. While carefully reviewing my claims records, I realized that one of my infertility treatment providers was double-billing my insurance company and me. Upon close inspection, I realized that my insurance company was paying the claim, and then my clinic was sending me a bill for the same services. The clinics billing statement did not show any evidence that my insurance company had already paid the bill.

It's important to look closely at all of your bills and EOBs. Your insurance company can have different fees negotiated with different doctors, and often the in-network providers are those who have agreed to the best fee structures. That's why you should always be careful to match your insurance coverage with your particular provider. You shouldn't necessarily assume your EOB has the right level of coverage. You need to be sure that coverage for your particular provider is correct. Also, there are codes that doctors and insurance companies use on EOBs to give brief explanations for what is covered and what is not covered. The same medical procedure can sometimes be entered using different codes, which can lead to coverage being denied when it shouldn't be. It's important to review your bills and EOBs closely, and ask questions.

In general, whenever you speak with anyone about billing, you should keep a thorough written record. This includes conversations with representatives of your insurance company, your doctor's office or clinic, or any business office which is handling your medical billing. You should note who you spoke to, when you spoke with this person, what his or her job title is, and who they are affiliated with. Be sure you accurately record the information they give you, and whether the information was verbal or written. Be specific about the bill or EOB you are inquiring about (using the date of service), and why you believe there is something wrong. Ask specific questions and be prepared to identify how you have confirmed that there may be a problem. If you have already attempted to negotiate your complaint with somebody else, be prepared to describe what this person's response was. Keep your own personal notes.

When I call somebody regarding an insurance bill I keep notes on the bill or attached to the bill. I have the proper records in front of me when I call, so I can make accurate references to costs, treatment procedures, or insurance claims. I write down the information I identified in the previous paragraph about who I am speaking with. I write down what my question was and what their response was. I also ask what time frame is required to address my problem. I confirm who will get back to me, and also how and when. When I get their answer on the phone, I sometimes ask them to send me their response to my question in writing. It is always good to have the information you request in writing, because that eliminates any disputes about who said what, and the information is not subject to interpretation. Getting a written response is always advisable in situations where exceptions are made or coverage is subject to interpretations.

Having spent some time processing health insurance claims myself I am somewhat familiar with these procedures. Calls are usually recorded these days, and it may also be helpful for you to know this. Recordings made as you speak to an insurance representative can be used to help clarify what you were and weren't told. When I worked doing disability claims, we actually did go back and review tapes with my supervisor when people claimed we said something we didn't.

Sometimes it is confusing to know who you need to contact. If you have gotten a bill that doesn't seem correct, then your medical provider is the place to start. If your question is about billing, ask to speak to someone in the business office. If you have a medical question, you may want to contact your doctor or nurse initially to determine what the next step might be. If you are not happy with the response you are getting from your medical or insurance provider, you can always request to speak with a supervisor. I also had experience working as a supervisor, and the supervisor always has more latitude and more expertise in handling questions or complaints.

If you are still not satisfied with the information you are given, you can inquire about appeal procedures. Find out who you can send an appeal to. Your appeal should be in writing but there may be specific documentation, records, or forms you need to submit. Sometimes your insurance booklet will have information on an appeals procedure. The supervisor should be able to tell you about an appeals procedure. A human resources person may also be able to assist you with this. Sometimes consulting a lawyer is advisable when approaching an appeals process and deciding the best approach to use.

When talking with your insurance company about a specific issue, try to get a time frame from them about when their processing will be completed. Ask for notification that actions are completed, and pay attention to these dates. Insurance companies often don't pay attention, letting time slip by, knowing that your opportunity to contest their coverage in the EOB will lapse. It's up to you to follow up on their commitments, and as Howard's story illustrates, sometimes you have to be very proactive to force coverage out of them. Sometimes, working with a single contact at the insurance company can be helpful. Try to get a call back extension or phone number from the person you are working with, so if you need to contact them again it will be easier to reach them directly.

My husband and I have had many claims initially denied. The reasons for denial can be as simple as your bills being sent to the wrong place, or as complicated as your clinic or doctor not forwarding your records or doing incomplete or inaccurate documentation. We were able to appeal and get coverage on many of these claims. You need to know how to appeal denials on your insurance claims. Different companies may have different procedures so be familiar with the process associated with your insurance benefit plan. Be sure to do the documentation I suggested above, and don't throw away any of this material. If you are not happy with the response you are getting, be sure to ask to speak with a supervisor. I was a supervisor and there were many problems I was able to work out to the satisfaction of the person filing the complaint. Talk to the supervisor about an action plan, outlining when and how things will happen, in what time frame and how you will be notified about it, and always request a written summary of this conversation.

You have the right to all of your medical records, and sometimes there may be incorrect information in those records. If incorrect information appears to be the nature of the problem in your claim denial, request a copy of your medical records so you have in hand exactly the same information as your insurance company. There may be a fee for these records to be copied, but it can be worth the money.

You should speak with your doctor if you find there are problems with your bills or medical records that continue to be unresolved. Often, there is something your doctor can do about it. It may mean that your doctor has to write a letter to your insurance company about your treatment, and list the reasons why you are or are not a candidate for a particular type of treatment. Find out what specific information the insurance company is asking for, before you approach your doctor's office. Many doctors are quite sophisticated in terms of dealing with insurance companies, and they know what to do to help you get the coverage you need.

An important strategy you can use when faced with an unfavorable insurance ruling is to ask your doctor to look at the ICD-9-CM diagnosis code that your doctor has used in your medical record. Every medical diagnosis has a special code that has three, four, or five digits assigned to it. This coding system helps an insurance company determine if your treatment is covered under your insurance plan. Sometimes, your symptoms, diagnosis or treatment can be entered under more than one of these codes. One code may be covered and another may not. Perhaps your doctor accidentally used the wrong code, while the charting was being done. That happened to me and it is easily corrected. Consult your doctor, if it appears your claim is being denied because of a diagnosis, and see if there is something your doctor can do to assist you. Sometimes, if your doctor submits the same medical procedures coded differently, you will get coverage.

Many of you will have coverage through a health maintenance organization (HMO). These plans generally do all of the billing work for you. This is obviously a great advantage, if you don't want to do that kind of paperwork. You should still save and review all paperwork to make sure everything was done correctly. Don't leave it to your insurance company to get it right—remember it's often your money on the line. Be sure to ask all of the questions outlined earlier regarding what type of treatment is covered. Also find out about their policy for defining a pre-existing condition, and whether there is a required wait time if you have a pre-existing condition. There also may be specific links between your HMO and the places you can get your medications, so inquire about that. The disadvantage of HMOs is that you must stay within their system of doctors and hospitals, and they may restrict your ability to get a second opinion, either inside or outside the HMO under your particular benefit plan.

PREPARING TO PAY THE BILL

Whether you have insurance or not, you need to be ready to pay the bills that inevitably go with fertility treatment. If you have insurance, you should try to anticipate which bills are going to be covered by your insurance, and at what percentage. Use your insurance benefit booklet as a guide. You don't want to be stuck with huge bills you didn't anticipate. Whether you have insurance or not, you should talk with your doctor or clinic representative and get a written estimate of what they anticipate your costs will be based on the treatment recommendations of your doctor. At least this way, you will have something in writing that shows their prediction of possible charges, and how they will be broken down. The authors of *The Fertility Book* have compiled a very helpful list, documenting what information you should request. It includes the following recommendations:

- Any administrative fees that they charge to start an IVF cycle.
- All professional service fees for the doctors overseeing your cycle. These fees should be broken down and listed individually.
- Charges for the evaluations and testing that will have to be done before your cycle starts. These should include HIV and hepatitis tests, CMV testing, semen analysis, and bacterial cultures.
- Ovulation-induction costs. These should include both drug and monitoring costs. Per test charges for blood testing and ultrasound should be detailed out with an estimate of the number of times they foresee doing these tests per cycle.
- Charges for stimulation with HCG.
- Cost of egg recovery. If it is to be done in a hospital setting any hospital charges that will be involved.
- Laboratory charges for IVF culturing. Micromanipulation if sperm injection is to be performed. The cost of assisted hatching, if that is to be performed.
- Fees for embryo freezing and storage.
- Embryo transfer fees. Again if this is to be done in a hospital setting, a list of anticipated hospital charges.
- Charges for any additional blood testing and monitoring of the luteal phase that they anticipate doing.(11)

Compiling all of this financial information may take a lot of time and energy, and at a time when you feel you have nothing left to give. Just the process of undergoing infertility treatment can be emotionally and physically draining. Sometimes, your partner can take on the burden of this vital role. You will have find that there are all kinds of new experiences you will have, while going on this journey, and some of them can be positive in ways you had not predicted. Being assertive many not be your normal style or behavior. At first, you may feel uncomfortable pushing these issues. However, when we commit to undergoing infertility treatment, we find ourselves saying and doing things we might not have considered before. After all, the financial stakes can be quite high.

Sue remembered how she took on this new role. "I think it made me have to view myself as a more assertive, aggressive person," she said. "That was…the part of me that I had to look at and question. It was the part—right there…my ability to assert myself. That was the heart of…my ability to change." Sue discovered that she was able to challenge and question information that was given to her. She just didn't accept everything that she was told on its face value. She was proactive about getting the right information regarding her infertility treatment.

Ann also talked about the ways she dealt with roadblocks during her treatment. "If I really needed to talk to my doctor and I couldn't get to him, that made me crazy. I would be at work, waiting to get phone calls, and they would come without information. I couldn't get the information quickly, and so I talked with him about it. I didn't want to call him at home. That felt intrusive. I didn't want to operate that way. It was boundaries. The things he wanted us to do didn't feel right." Ann previously had mentioned the problems she had with the support staff in her doctor's office. At times, she also had problems with getting medical questions answered by her doctor in a timely and appropriate manner.

Without getting good answers to questions, it is difficult to approach your insurance company regarding problems with claims and billing. This can be a huge source of frustration. If you can't put the medical bills and claims information together in a meaningful way, then you cannot be certain that you are getting the insurance benefits you are entitled to get. Often, you need to be assertive and proactive in pursuit of resolution. You should not spend any additional money out of your pocket unless you are sure you have to. Sue and Ann both were able to take control at times when they knew in their hearts things didn't feel right. Trust yourself. Rely on what you are feeling and thinking. Talk about it with your partner, your doctor, or friends and family. Money issues should be clearly resolved, and you should not rely on inconsistent explanations. If you have questions, pursue them persistently. Claims people often come up with reasons that mistakes are "right," instead of finding the error and correcting it.

Another way to be proactive is to actively pursue understanding of your medications. You may be able to find a pharmacy or drug company that specializes in infertility treatment. I did and I found this incredibly helpful. They knew the importance of timeliness for certain medications, and would even have my medications delivered to me at my office, just hours after we had spoken, in cases when time was critical. They also could give me additional information about my medications. My representative was very professional and knew about insurance coverage. She was able to use her expertise to help me get the medications I needed, and she also saved me money. Before you sign up, be sure to verify that the specific drug provider is covered under your insurance plan. My representative got her company added to the preferred provider list under my insurance, so that all of my medications were covered at the higher, in-network rate. This resulted in a substantial savings to me. This was not the result of luck; it was the result of assertiveness. I discussed this possibility with her, and she was able to make it happen.

Insurance coverage can make a big difference in the cost of your infertility treatment. In most states, no coverage is mandated, and you will often have to bear the expense on your own. Even with insurance, your portion of the costs can be substantial. Infertility treatment is not cheap. There are also many clinics and programs that offer brochures and information about loan and financing programs for people who need financial assistance to undergo infertility treatment. I have heard stories of people who have placed themselves in serious financial debt during their infertility journey.

You should reserve some time to think about and discuss financial planning as another component of your infertility treatment. If you are a person who tends to have difficulty with money management and balancing your checkbook, infertility treatment can be a real danger zone for you, because the bills can seem to mount endlessly. Adoption can also easily cost $20,000. The stress of this financial strain can ultimately place stress on your relationship with your partner.

Different people have different ideas about money management, and how much can be reasonably spent. You both need to agree on how much you are able and willing to spend in your quest to have a child. It is a reality we all must come to terms with. Money is the number one reason that marriages fail. When money problems are combined with not having children, this can place enormous pressure on the people involved, and on their relationship. Paradoxically, the pressure caused by money problems can also negatively impact your infertility treatment.

Medical providers are very aware that the costs are escalating and that there are patients who are unable to pay their bills. Some of these healthcare providers are trying to come up with some creative ways to assist people who need medical treatment and are on a tighter budget. Some clinics require upfront money and offer loans. Be sure you understand both the costs involved and the likelihood of needing more than one round of treatment. Requiring upfront money has become very common. Taking out loans to pay upfront can add to the costs, and decrease your ability to pursue a second round of treatment.

There is a growing trend where some clinics ask you to pay upfront money when you begin your treatment but then guarantee you a refund on a portion of this money, if your treatment is not successful. This is for people in a situation where no insurance coverage is available. This is a welcome change for people undergoing infertility treatment, who are facing the prospect of enormous bills. It is so frustrating when you have a limited amount of money, and you pay for treatment that is not successful. Often, you find you don't have enough money for the next treatment. You can have a lingering feeling that, if you only had enough money, you would eventually hit upon the treatment that would get you pregnant. These are the kinds of money problems that can add stress to the infertility journey, and potentially impact its outcome.

Sometimes expensive fertility treatments give you an opportunity to deduct a portion of their cost from your income taxes. You may be able to get tax benefits if your medical bills are of a certain size in relation to your income. You will need to have all of your billing and payment records to document costs for income tax purposes. If you have very high medical bills and insurance costs, consult someone who is knowledgeable about taxes. You may be able to get tax benefits from the cumulative amount of your medical expenses.

THE IMPORTANCE OF BEING PROACTIVE AND TAKING CONTROL

My husband and I felt it would be very useful to share our own insurance story with you. Our experience with insurance companies and infertility treatment highlights how the system works, or doesn't work, and the potential pitfalls that can arise for those of us caught in the middle. In our example, we will share some steps that we took to ensure we got as much coverage as we could from our insurance company. We hope our experience can help guide you through your insurance maze.

After we decided on our course of treatment with our doctor, the clinic provided us with a detailed estimate of costs. Initially, we anticipated having very little, or no insurance coverage for fertility treatments. Like many couples, we were asked to put up a large amount of money before we started our infertility treatment. In our case, this upfront money was close to $20,000. This is part of why they gave us such a detailed initial estimate of our costs.

Healthcare providers like to have upfront money. They are well aware that many insurance companies don't cover fertility treatment, or that they tend to process claims very slowly. Insurance reimbursement can be a long, drawn out process. Many claims are contested for a variety of reasons, and they have to be processed multiple times. With upfront money, your healthcare provider can "take payment" right away. Here's how it works. Once you receive some type of healthcare service, a bill is sent to you and to your insurance carrier. Then, while your claim is being processed, the healthcare provider takes "payment" from your upfront money. This money is only returned to your account after your insurance makes payment.

As I explained earlier, initial medical billing is almost always over-charged. Your insurance company likely has negotiated service rates with your provider, but in our case, the infertility clinic would bill us the full amount, without the cost reduction, and take this amount from our upfront money. This was customary practice when we underwent treatment, and many providers continue to follow this pattern. The costs are "adjusted" later by the insurance company, but in the interim the clinic takes your money.

Having money tied up in the healthcare system is challenging. Reimbursement is incredibly slow, and the reality is that they (your clinic and your insurance company) want to hold onto your money as long as they can. In our case, the clinic would receive a letter from our insurance company with the adjusted fee amount, and they would not be quick about returning that money to us. They would keep the full payment on their books, even though that portion of our "budget" had been paid and adjusted. Then, our insurance company would send them money on top of the money we had initially given our infertility clinic. When I carefully reviewed our claims statements, I realized money was being sent to my infertility clinic, and we were not being reimbursed by the clinic. Since we had paid the bill already, the reimbursement from the insurance company could have come to us. I promptly contacted my insurance company, and had the payments redirected to me. This was better than sending the money to our clinic, and then having to wait for them to adjust the bill and reimburse me.

On numerous occasions I spoke with the business staff at my infertility clinic, and asked them to send me all of the billing information. I wanted to cross reference their records regarding my treatment, the costs, and what was reimbursed through the insurance company. They repeatedly told me it would be done, and then did not follow through. While all this was going on, I was not aware of the fact that my infertility clinic had filed for bankruptcy. It was only after I found out they had filed for bankruptcy, that I finally received a printout from the infertility clinic. It was incredibly difficult to decipher, because they just sent me a computer print out with codes and numbers on it, and nothing else to specifically define the nature of the treatment. It was very long and poorly put together.

I was familiar with some of the codes, and I used our EOB records to cross reference fees and dates. By doing this, I could make some sense out of what we had been billed, and what was owed to us.

We were able to come up with documentation showing what the infertility clinic owed us, and we were able to get some reimbursement. I have to say that this required me to be extremely proactive. I expended a lot of time and energy reviewing these records, and I let my clinic know that I was well aware of what was going on with the billing. If I hadn't done all this, I am quite certain we would not have received any money back. It was an important lesson for us.

As it was, we lost some of our upfront money in the bankruptcy of our clinic. Had we ensured that insurance reimbursements came directly to us from the beginning, the clinic would not have received any "double payments" (as they did), and most of the money owed to us would have come back from the insurance company. While these circumstances are unusual, it does serve to illustrate how attentive you should be to issues around money. Understanding how the system works is the first step in becoming proactive, and being proactive helps to ensure you get the maximum coverage you can at the minimum cost. I hope our example can help empower you to take charge and get knowledge of your insurance and how the billing and reimbursement works.

CHAPTER 6
LEGAL ISSUES

The world of collaborative reproductive technology has opened up unimaginable possibilities for those of us who had little hope of having a child. Collaborative reproduction is when a couple uses donor gametes from another person. In the case of a surrogate, the surrogate agrees to carry and give birth to the child. Collaborative reproduction has also opened up a "Pandora's Box" in terms of the complex legal relationships that arise in this new world of infertility treatment. The new reproductive technology has offered us sperm and egg donors, surrogates, embryos, and frozen embryos. We now have open adoptions and international adoptions that occur on a regular basis. The complexity of the legal relationships that can occur as a result of these new infertility and adoption opportunities is also quite astounding.

I recently heard a news report about a woman who created embryos using her eggs and her husband's sperm. These embryos were frozen while she was married. Later, she and her husband got divorced. After the divorce, without her husband's knowledge, she forged his signature and went back to the clinic and had the embryos transferred. She was successful and had a child, and then she decided to sue her husband for child support.

Our infertility clinic had a case where a woman and man came in and said they were married. They had infertility treatment and had a child together. The clinic later learned they had lied and that he was married to another woman. His wife eventually did file litigation against the clinic.

People who choose to donate eggs and sperm usually do not have any idea who ultimately uses the donated eggs and sperm. The resulting child may have many biological siblings that he or she is unaware of having. In seminars I have attended, we have talked about the possibility that two people descended from the same donor might meet and fall in love, while unknowingly being biologically related.

You may have heard about a sister who volunteered to be a surrogate for her sister who was unable to have a child. When you think about it you realize that in a way she is both that child's aunt and the mother. There are not always laws available that address some of these multiple, complex relationships. The legal, emotional, and psychological ramifications of these complex situations need special, careful consideration for everybody who is involved.

I talked earlier about how the legal and ethical worlds have not caught up with the medical and technological worlds in many instances. This is an ongoing challenge.

Many questions that arise during collaborative reproduction do not have legal answers in place yet. A recent surrogacy case serves as a perfect example of this. A couple, unable to bear a child of their own, engaged a surrogate to carry their baby. During the course of her pregnancy, the future parents decided that the pregnancy should be terminated. There is currently no law in place to dictate what should happen. Does the surrogate have any right to protect the baby she is carrying? What if there are medical problems with the baby? What if the parents are getting divorced or one of them is terminally ill? There are so many contingencies and no laws in place to govern them yet.

There are many other examples where these situations can arise with new infertility treatments. Would-be parents choose a course of action which is newly developed in order to have a child, but it has no legal mandate to govern it, no precedent in law. Cases are being addressed and laws are beginning developed, but this is an evolving process. Just because a law is applicable in one state doesn't mean it is applicable in other states, and appeals are ongoing. Hopefully with time there will be more legal guidelines available.

The variety of infertility solutions pursued today can raise many complex legal issues. Frankly, this was something my husband and I had not even thought about before we started our treatment. In retrospect we should have given legal issues more consideration. At one point our clinic put a stack of papers in front of us to sign, and you would have thought it was a real estate closing. Having gone through the process, my bias is to recommend that you do see an attorney when sorting out the legal issues related to certain types of infertility treatment.

One of the things I learned working as a social worker in hospitals is that the advancement of technology and medical knowledge is really astounding. We see that today in the rapidly advancing world of infertility treatment. I became equally aware that, as these wonderful medical breakthroughs occur, the ethical and legal approaches to these treatments do not advance at the same rate. Most hospitals now have some sort of ethicist or ethical group that reviews cases and the complex issues that can arise from these new technological breakthroughs. I participated in an ethics group at one of Chicago's major teaching hospitals in the past. You quickly realize there are no easy solutions and rarely definite right or wrong answers to these multifaceted questions. Cases need to be reviewed on their individual merits.

We have already discussed the fact that new types of infertility treatments are here, and more are coming in the near future. Our doctors and scientists continue to gain knowledge and experience, stretching treatment into new areas of possibility. As a result, laws and regulations are unable to keep up with the legal and ethical questions that arise regularly in hospitals. There are very few laws governing how to evaluate situations where a donor or a surrogate is used. Cases are beginning to be tried in the courts. Currently the governing body that deals with these questions within the medical profession is the American Society of Assisted Reproductive Medicine. It is important to note that what they say is not the law, but simply their recommendations about ethics and legal compliance. They have the broadest and most up-to-date knowledge about the world of infertility treatment.

INSURANCE AND THE LAW

Laws governing insurance regulation are highly variable today, and this can directly impact treatment choices and cost to you. As I highlighted earlier, Eliza and Todd and Sue and Howard had very different expenses and outcomes, and much of this was based on their insurance coverage. The New England Journal of Medicine addressed the issue of how laws impact insurance and treatment choices in an article, published in Volume 347, August 29, 2002, by Dr. Tarun Jain, MD, and Bernard Harlow. This 2002 article looked specifically at insurance and IVF outcomes. The results of their study were reviewed in Hope, the Illinois Chapter of RESOLVE's quarterly magazine, Volume 24, 2002. Hope found that: "Although most insurance companies in the United States do not cover IVF, a few states…mandate this coverage. The authors used 1998 data reported to the Center for Disease Control and Prevention...by 360 fertility clinics...and 2000 United States Census data to determine utilization and outcomes of IVF services based on the status of the insurance coverage."(12) The study found that "clinics in the few states that required complete coverage performed more IVF cycles than clinics in states where only partial or no coverage was required."(13) The study also showed that "state mandated insurance coverage for IVF service is associated with increased utilization of these services and...decreases in the number of embryos transferred per cycle, the percentage of cycles resulting in pregnancy, and the percentage of pregnancies with three or more fetuses."(14)

This study reveals that coverage is often driven by state law, and that, when there is coverage, it changes the choices made by patients undergoing IVF. Not all states that mandated infertility insurance coverage of some kind had the same coverage for IVF. In those states mandating complete coverage, there were more IVF cycles done and this was directly connected to the state laws regarding infertility treatment. In those states where women had real choice, they chose to transfer fewer embryos in order to reduce their odds of having multiple births and ending up with twins and triplets. They made this choice, even though it reduced their odds of having a successful pregnancy. In states where women and their families bore the costs, they chose to transfer a greater number of embryos to increase their odds of a successful pregnancy, and so reduce the potential number of IVF transfers necessary (and limit the costs). These are difficult trade-offs to weigh, but women appear to decide differently when given a choice that is not driven by cost.

There is a great deal of advocacy around state laws today. The study cited above found that in 1998 "only three states required complete insurance coverage and only five states required partial coverage."(15) More state legislatures are currently considering adopting state laws in these areas today, and the legal situation is changing constantly. Laws still vary from state to state regarding infertility insurance coverage. The laws are also changing because they are continually facing legal challenges. For these reasons, I do not want to write about specific states or their laws. If I did, the information might be obsolete by the time you read this book. Many states remain reluctant to mandate that insurance carriers cover infertility treatment because of the costs. Insurance providers will sometimes pull out of states where regulations are perceived as too costly, reducing the competition within the state, which eventually can cause costs to rise even more.

Here's a list of states that currently have some type of law that governs infertility insurance: Illinois, Montana, Ohio, Maryland, Arkansas, New York, Hawaii, West Virginia, Rhode Island, and Massachusetts. Other states may have laws that force insurance companies to offer some type of infertility coverage, such as California. You can find out the specifics of the state you live in and current law by consulting your local RESOLVE Chapter. RESOLVE's address can be found in Chapter 22. A local attorney who specializes in infertility legal issues can also shed some light on the laws in your state.

In light of the vast expense and often limited benefit packages offered by insurance carriers, people and their doctors will often choose the treatment that is covered under their benefit plan. However, this may not be the most appropriate or medically indicated treatment. It may not have the highest success rate, either.

Sue and Howard's treatment reflects the power of insurance companies. Sue described how her insurance company's guidelines required her to undergo unnecessary treatment. They knew that their insemination cycles had a very low probability of success, but in order to have coverage for other procedures they were required to comply with the treatment guidelines. Todd also discussed the challenges and anxiety of dealing with insurance issues. In his experience, the insurance company "was so incredibly difficult that the fertility doctors, wherever possible, were trying to prescribe things so that it would maximize [the] insurance company's possibility of covering a small piece of it."

In many instances, the reality is that fertility treatment would be less costly to society if the law required insurance companies to offer more comprehensive coverage. If there was less restricted coverage, doctors would not have to order unnecessary treatment, as they did in

Sue's case. They could go straight to the appropriate treatment and save money and ultimately have the best shot at the most desirable outcomes. They also wouldn't waste so much time and money contesting claims, as they did with Todd's doctors.

If you feel you are entitled to insurance coverage or reimbursement that you aren't getting, you can always make an appeal. Sometimes this can be done more effectively with the help of a lawyer. You can seek legal advice with attorneys that specialize in areas of infertility. However, before you contact an attorney about insurance claims denials, make sure you know whether your insurance plan is self-insured or a traditional indemnity insurance plan. This will help your lawyer know how to proceed. If you don't know what type of insurance plan you have, contact your human resources department or go directly to your insurance company to get this information. Depending on your state's laws, self-insured businesses may not need to comply. Often, a human resources representative or an insurance claims representative can give you helpful ideas and information about how to fight denials of insurance claims or discrimination in your workplace.

In my home state of Illinois, we have a Department of Insurance. The purpose of this Department is to protect the rights of insurance consumers under the Illinois Insurance code and other insurance specific legislation. They are a watchdog agency for all of the licensed insurance companies in the state of Illinois. Healthcare consumers are free to contact them and register complaints about a licensed insurance agent, broker, or company that the consumer believes has not complied with Illinois regulation. You should check in your local area to see if a similar consumer advocacy department is available to you. Before you call a consumer protection agency, make sure you have all the necessary information prepared. Write down the names of the people you spoke with at your insurance company, your human resources department, or any state agency you have had previous contact with. Be ready to share this information, including what they have told you, and be prepared with specific questions. Take written notes on what you are told, by whom, and be sure to note the date and time of this conversation with any state agency.

Beyond state laws, there are some federal legal precedents being set. In June of 1998, there was a case sent before the United States Supreme Court that directly impacted insurance coverage for people undergoing infertility treatment. The case was *Bragdon v Abbott*. In this case, a woman who was positive for HIV filed a lawsuit against her dentist because he would not treat her due to her HIV status. Her lawyer filed legal action under the American with Disabilities Act. How does this relate to infertility treatment? What happened was the court determined that, to get protection against discrimination, a person must have "a physical or mental impairment that substantially limits one or more major life activities." In her case, the court defined reproduction as a major life activity. The argument, of course, is that infertility is a physical impairment that, by definition, limits the major life activity of reproduction. According to this decision, infertility can be viewed as a disability.

While I was going through infertility treatment, I learned about a female police officer here in Chicago who sued the city because she could not get insurance coverage for infertility treatment. The basis of her case was that infertility is a disability under the Americans with Disabilities Act. The federal court upheld this interpretation. The city settled the case with her. I thought about pursuing this legal option myself, when I first learned I would not have insurance coverage. What you have to decide is whether you believe that infertility is indeed a disability. You should realize there are no guarantees for you, if you choose to go down this long, legal road. You should know that, even if you win, the decision may be appealed. This is another legal tool, though, and the good news is that the Supreme Court ruling gives us reason to be optimistic regarding future cases. One day, refusal to cover the costs of infertility treatment may be definitively ruled discriminatory under law.

We should all be watching developments in the law closely, as they will be changing rapidly. More and more people are becoming active in pushing for changes in the law. Family law is a hot topic right now, and many new regulations protecting the rights of families are being written every day. This is another way that you can become proactive and empowered in your infertility journey. You can find out about changing laws and legal advocacy groups by joining RESOLVE or participating in their programming. You too can join with others and become a public advocate for laws that protect the interests of people like us who just want the best shot at becoming parents. Why shouldn't the law help protect our pursuit of this "major life activity"?

CONSENT IN THE NEW LEGAL REALM

Many new legal issues are being addressed around the world in many different ways. Countries like Austria, Denmark, the United Kingdom, Sweden, and Norway have established national regulation of the legal status of oocyte, or egg, donations. Some countries such as Austria prohibit all egg donations, including commercial egg donations. Other countries, such as Canada, have legislation in place that legally allows the donor to be voluntary and anonymous. At a recent conference I learned there are places in Europe and Australia where laws guarantee that a child conceived with the help of a donor can have full access to the donor records when they turn 18. As you can see, there are many different legal approaches to these issues, and as new laws and regulations are written in the U.S., they will likely vary significantly from state to state.

My purpose in reviewing these legal issues is to help you ask the right questions in relation to the specific types of infertility treatment you are planning to pursue. I cannot tell you what all the laws are where you live because each state is different and these laws are constantly being revised and reviewed. I can give you some questions to raise with your clinic and attorney. You should be aware that there are many legal issues out there, many of which relate to future anonymity and the availability of information. In many cases, this has to do with what your future child will be able to know about their origins. Always keep in mind that standards of practice can change from state to state.

Standards for screening donors, for example, are quite variable. If you go out of state for an egg donor the law in that state may differ from your home state. Sue and Howard discussed this issue with me. "We had our egg donation done in California," Howard said, "and the contract had to show that the egg donor couldn't come back and claim the baby...Going out of state is trickier because every state has different laws, so you have to know which state is going to be friendlier to the donee, to us recipients."

Sue added: "I would get a lawyer who is really experienced. In our case this lawyer was not... You can't read those contracts by yourself. Not the egg donor stuff. But when you go for the IVF there is stuff in there about what if you have frozen eggs, what are you going to do with them? The third party stuff got pretty complicated and I don't think we could have understood it ourselves. It was a ten page contract."

When my husband and I decided to do an egg donor procedure, they handed us a thick stack of papers and asked us to sign documents. Some of these documents related to what we would do with any extra embryos we had, and how long they would be stored. No one had prepared us for considering these complex questions. We were given virtually no information about what was in these papers either beforehand or when they were handed to us. My husband and I asked all of the questions we could think of at the time. Your doctor is supposed to give you all the pertinent information regarding your treatment before you sign these documents, and by signing them you confirm that this was done. In our case, we had not been given any specific information that could help us determine what to do about these potential frozen embryos. If our treatment was successful, we could have many more frozen embryos than we would ever transfer.

At the time, I was so overwhelmed with the idea of having this fertility treatment that I was unable to give these questions the proper time and attention they deserved. My husband and I should have had a long discussion about these issues before the papers were in front of us to sign. As it was, we were in agreement, but these complex questions are not necessarily easily resolved with your partner. We went ahead, after our doctor told us that we would have to make some type of final decision within five years, once we stored our embryos. We had to put our faith in the clinic we were working with and trust that what they were having us sign was in our best interest and the best interest of the frozen embryos. We would've been better served to ask for all these documents in advance, so that we had adequate time to review and discuss them together. Then, if necessary, we could have also consulted our attorney.

There are always consent forms and documents that you will be asked to sign no matter what type of infertility treatment you will undertake. This is obviously true for adoption as well. There is often little, if any, information given ahead of time to help you understand and sort out all of this paperwork. By the time they are asking you to sign, it is usually such a high-stress moment already that you may be inclined to simply sign these documents without reviewing them. There are some questions you can raise when you are presented with this information. Diane Clapp, BSN, RN outlines them in an article called: "Questions to Ask When Signing Consent Forms or Contracts." It can be found in the 2002 spring issue of *Family Building* magazine. These questions can serve as a roadmap for you, when you are asked to sign consent forms or contracts in these circumstances. They include the following:

- Ask for clarification if you have questions about wording used in the form.
- When possible, have a third party (spouse, friend, lawyer, etc.) review any forms before you sign them.
- Ask how long a period of time the signed consent documentation will be applicable.
- Use a pen, not pencil, to complete forms.
- Answer all relevant questions; do not leave any questions blank. If a question is not relevant to your situation, write "na" (not applicable).
- Write your initials beside any changes made, for example, if you delete a word or phrase in the original document.
- Always date the form when you sign it.
- Ask for a copy of the consent form or contract for your own records.
- If you are signing a consent form for an assisted reproductive technology procedure, request in writing what the clinic agrees to do financially if the cycle is cancelled.
- Ask if the clinic has a policy regarding storage and transfer of gametes (sperm) or embryos to other facilities either in or out of state. Sign and date any statements relating to this policy.(16)

Reviewing your consent forms carefully is another way for you to take a more active role in your treatment. Ask for forms in advance, and do not hesitate to voice any concerns you have at this key moment in your infertility journey. Be prepared to sign forms, either as they are, or as you wish to amend them. No one wants legal issues to delay their treatment, but careful thought beforehand can be critical to the future.

The reality is that doctors and clinics are focused on the ways to help you get pregnant successfully. They are not thinking about legal issues or the stress and confusion these documents might cause you. They generally do not take the time to explain these documents and their meaning of their content to you. For them, these papers are a legal formality of going forward with treatment. You will have to ask specific questions to get them to take the time to explain the documents. Often, these papers are presented by a nurse, who may have little knowledge of their legal ramifications (though some nurses are quite knowledgeable and helpful). Everyone feels a sense of urgency to get this paperwork signed quickly and get to the treatment phase as soon as possible. The goal after all is to have a baby, not birth a contract. Yet, signing these papers often represents entering into a contract that will be binding on the future. Knowing what you are signing up for is critical for you, even if your clinic treats it as pro forma.

CRITICAL LEGAL AREAS TO REVIEW

There are a number of major areas where getting legal advice can be very important. One is when you decide to use an egg or sperm donor. It doesn't matter if the donor is known or is anonymous. All donations should be subject to clear, legal agreements. When this involves an egg donor, the agreement will cover your obligations to pay her medical expenses and compensation, if any. It will also establish limitations on the donor's future rights with regard to any embryos or children that result from your treatment. In terms of donor insemination (sperm donation) the laws are usually fairly straightforward and basically say that the donor has no rights. The husband of the woman carrying the child is the father. Laws governing sperm or egg donations generally don't designate any legal differences between an anonymous and a known donor.

The laws regarding the screening of egg and sperm donors differ from state to state, so be sure to get clarification regarding this area. You should feel assured that your potential anonymous donors have been well-screened, and that the background materials you are given, which include their family medical histories, are accurate. In either type of donation, egg or sperm donor insemination, when the donor is known it is really important to have a legal agreement in place, even if the donor is a friend or family member. It is also important that both you and the donor have separate legal representation, so that all parties have a complete understanding of the agreement.

All of these same injunctions hold true for surrogacy, too. If anything, surrogacy should be governed by more carefully crafted agreements. In many cases, there is no law or legal precedent that will apply, and so the contract you create with your surrogate will dictate much of your legal standing. This contract involves so much more than what you will pay them, and should include clear language on how decisions are made during pregnancy, what rights the surrogate will have after birth, and can include the future rights of your child to have contact with their birth mother. These are highly complex issues, and the legal ramifications will vary from state to state, so a lawyer with particular experience in this area of the law is essential. Once again, having these agreements in place is critical, even if your surrogate is a friend or a family member.

Legal agreements and representation are a mandatory part of any adoption procedure. Different states have different laws about the amount of time the birth mother has to change her mind about the adoption. Some people choose to have an adoption where the birth mother remains an ongoing presence in the child's life. There may be agreements made about how often she can see the child and ways in which she can communicate. These agreements should all be put in writing so that they become binding. This protects all concerned parties. It is also important to remember that paid leave for adoption is not readily available at this time. Different companies may have different policies about it, but there are currently no laws in place regarding this. Again get clarification from the company you are with regarding their policies on leave. It is helpful to get this in writing.

Embryo donation is another specific area where it is critical to investigate legal issues and have written agreements. You must make sure that any legal agreement is signed by the father and the mother on both sides. This avoids any potential legal battles in the future. Sometimes it is difficult to track down the father and mother in the future, if questions arise, so be sure to have everything spelled out in the written agreement. This will be money well spent.

Whenever you engage in collaborative reproduction, there are additional complex legal issues. Make sure you are familiar with the laws of your state and those of the state where you are having your infertility treatment done. In cases where anonymous egg donors are used, they are often recruited by clinics. Their consent agreements may be with these clinics or other infertility related programs. There are some states that may be friendlier to specific infertility procedures than others. Local reproductive endocrinologists, specialized lawyers, or reproductive health clinics can be the best sources for this information where you live. If you have doubts about the legal information you are given, be sure to find an attorney who specializes in the law regarding assisted reproductive technologies or adoption, depending on your needs. Both adoption and infertility-treatment require legal specialization.

Many things can happen during the course of infertility treatment and during the course of a pregnancy. Contingencies need to be spelled out in writing. For example if a surrogate decides she doesn't want to continue with the pregnancy, what will happen? If additional, unexpected medical expenses arise for the donor or surrogate, how will that issue be addressed? In the case of a woman who has frozen embryos and wants to have a second child, what if the man decides he does not want to use them? Many people recommend counseling, or at least a psychological examination, for the donor and the people who want to have the child. In some programs this is mandatory. Who will do this assessment and how will it be paid for? What happens if there is a divorce or a death? Make sure you have legal documents that are very clear regarding the financial pieces of these many complex relationships. Payments should relate to treatment and services needed to ensure the best possible environment to produce a healthy child.

You should also have a clear understanding about what donor information you are legally entitled to have, and what additional information you would like to request. What information will you get about the genetic, medical, psychological and substance abuse histories of your potential donors? Be sure to ask how many generations back this information will go, and whether this information is genuine and reliable. Donor generated statements are not necessarily reliable, and your clinic should have a screening process. In the case of a surrogate mother, you should consider what safeguards are in place to ensure she maintains a healthy regime while pregnant. What happens if she does not comply with this? Make sure the relevant issues are put out there for discussion with all parties, and that your legal agreement covers everything possible. We have all heard about cases where things backfired, because the legal work wasn't in place. The consequences of this can be devastating for all concerned. Make sure the issue of disposition of extra embryos is addressed in your legal paperwork. These safeguards protect you, the genetic parents, and the potential child or children that may come from this arrangement.

If, after talking with your attorney, you discover there are legal problems related to your infertility treatment, make sure you discuss this with your doctor, embryologist, or other appropriate person at your clinic. You and your attorney can meet with the doctor, if necessary, to try and sort out these specifics in the paperwork you will be signing. Your doctor should be willing to work with your attorney under these circumstances.

There can be negative consequences, if you are not aware of the legal issues associated with the adoption process or infertility treatment you choose. You need to make sure that all of the proper legal mechanisms are in place to protect you, your partner, and your child. Consulting somebody with legal expertise and carefully thinking about the legal ramifications of the infertility choices you make is a critical element in this process. This knowledge and expertise are mechanisms that can empower and protect you in terms of your "foreseeable future interests." The ethical considerations are closely intertwined with the legal ones. In the future, your child may desire access to all of the information possible to determine his or her origins, and this is both a legal and ethical question that needs to be carefully thought out and provided for now. There are many other "foreseeable future interests" to sort out. What would be the legal and ethical consequences for you, your partner, and child in the event of a divorce? There may be particular custody questions that need identification and clarification in cases of collaborative reproduction. Or another example would be: how will future disagreements around the fate of frozen embryos be decided?

THE "LAW" OF UNINTENDED CONSEQUENCES

Every case of collaborative reproduction will have its own ethical and legal peculiarities. In our own case, we signed a mountain of papers when we initiated our infertility treatment. Among the papers my husband and I signed was a document saying that our child would not have any access to information regarding who her donor was. This was the only option we were given at our infertility clinic. Our decision closed the door on our daughter's ability to acquire any additional information about her donor that she might want to obtain some time in the future. We hope that our decision is something she will understand and be okay with if it comes up some day in the future.

Donors have rights, too, and one important right for many of them is this future privacy. Our daughter shares this right with her donor, which we decided was probably the best thing. But legal agreements can sometimes have unintended consequences, and ours precludes our daughter and the donor from ever waiving their legal rights to privacy. They might both be willing to do so at some point in the future, but they would have no way of pursuing information about or contacting one-another. It is important to remember that binding legal agreements are critical in cases of collaborative reproduction and adoption, but that protective limitations can sometimes cut both ways. The question of origins can be profound and personal, whatever the law or a contract says.

We didn't seem to have much choice when we signed our papers, and we hoped that this arrangement would create some "closure" around the issue. But, like many things, this is something impossible to foresee. Remember this when you consider the many limitations your legal agreements will necessarily create. Because the laws remain hazy in many of these emerging areas, it is important to establish your present and future rights through a good contract. You should protect yourself and your potential child with a well-crafted legal agreement. But remember, the more rigorous this legal agreement is, the less future flexibility there will be. If this is a concern to you, be sure to talk with your lawyer about it—especially if there is a particular part of the agreement that doesn't seem right to you. Pro forma legal documents are often used, and these can be amended. But you should only do this with professional legal advice. The other parties in your contract will have to agree, and this isn't always possible.

Exploring and resolving legal issues in advance is always advisable. Being legally uninformed and unprotected is a way to get burned. Being proactive about understanding legal issues is critical, and taking the time to acquire the necessary knowledge can be empowering. You should be comfortable with the legal agreements you make, even if, at times, you know there are potential future consequences that can result. Only you can weigh these factors and make the decisions that are right for you. A good lawyer will help you understand the trade-offs, but fundamentally the decision should be yours. The legal agreements you make will both protect and bind you, and your potential child, in the future. Make your legal commitments consciously, knowing that they will give you both rights and limitations, and that these may potentially have unintended future consequences.

CHAPTER 7
MAKING THE DECISION TO STOP TREATMENT

When I thought about writing this book I knew it was imperative to include a chapter on people choosing to stop treatment. That is one of the reasons I wanted to interview Ann. For some people, stopping treatment is a difficult decision, which gets put off for a long time. Other people experience a relatively short infertility journey and know in their hearts that stopping treatment is the best choice for them. Making the decision to stop infertility treatment is what this chapter is about. This decision can be a conscious choice, but knowing how to arrive at this decision and still feel all right about stopping treatment is challenging. Yet, making this choice is, in fact, another way to gain control over the infertility issues that we face. It is a viable option, if difficult to choose. We live in a world where we are invited to attend baby showers, and where one of the first questions people ask when you get married is, "What about children?" It is often a painful process to get to the point where you say, "I can't do this treatment anymore."

When people first learn they have infertility problems, they often set off on the road of infertility treatment and do what they can to have children. This pursuit often becomes an all-consuming part of their lives. Eliza talked about this with me when she said, "It becomes addictive. It really becomes addictive. This doesn't work and let me move to the next treatment. It is totally addictive."

Her husband, Todd, echoed the notion that it is easy to get on board the train and try everything you possibly can to have a child. His response to hearing Eliza's statement was: "As hard as it is, you know it is such an emotional issue. You really have to keep your head straight. Listen very carefully to the doctors as to what your chances are. Make an assessment based on how much money you have and what the probabilities are. Figure out what makes the most sense. I think people get so wrapped up in this, and the odds of them being able to conceive are really so small. And yet you can burn through an insane amount of money and not even get pregnant. I think you have to have a mental stop point in mind, when you say that if it doesn't happen at this point…you have to accept reality, and look into adoption or being a childless couple."

I spoke with Ann at length about stopping treatment, since she had chosen not to have children. In her case, her husband had gotten seriously ill when she was involved in infertility treatment, and she wanted to devote her full attention and energy toward helping him get through his medical problems. Her reason for stopping was external. She said: "Everything looked different, my entire perspective changed. I don't know how I would have stopped. I would have eventually stopped. I was trying to get close to the place to stop when he got sick. I have a lot of healthy respect for the trouble with ending treatment."

In addition to her personal experience with infertility, Ann also works with others who have infertility issues and may be grappling with stopping treatment. I asked her to elaborate for me on some of the personal and professional guidelines she used for herself and with others. "I say we all have our limits," Ann told me. "Nobody can tell us what they are. It is something we have to figure out for ourselves. Essentially we weren't meant to exhaust all of our resources to become mothers, fathers, and parents. You want to be sure you have something left over when it is all over. It costs a lot. Finances are not the biggest part. It is the costs to your emotions, your relationships, your friendships. It isn't good for us to be willing to pay that."

It is so hard to let go of the dream of having a child when you and your partner have put so much of yourselves into the effort. We make sacrifices physically, medically, emotionally, financially, and in our relationships. Personal sacrifices are compounded by those we often make to go on working. Ann alluded to sacrifices in relationships in her statements, and perhaps these have also occurred in your case. Sometimes those of us trying to have a child feel we have to put some distance between ourselves and other people. This can be particularly true when the other people have children or are family members who don't understand the difficult struggles we are enduring in infertility. Expressing your struggles to others can feel like an additional burden. Then, when you get to a place where you might consider stopping treatment, the natural inclination is to look back over all of the difficult sacrifices you have made up to that point. It can be very hard to let go. How do you come to be reconciled with that decision and find comfort in your own heart and mind?

We have spoken a lot about the roller coaster ride that infertility treatment can be for us. In treatment, we explore all of the available technological options in our quest to have a child. Eventually, we get to the point where we recognize that these alternatives may not be likely to work for us. When you find you are having multiple treatment failures, it is crucial to sit down with your doctor and have a frank discussion. You need to ask why he or she believes your treatment is not working, and find out what recommendations he or she has for any additional treatment for you. You should clearly understand the success rates associated with these infertility treatments given your specific situation, and find out if your doctor recommends that you continue along this path. Your doctor may recommend, or you may come to feel, that this is the time and place to stop treatment. While making this decision may seem right to you, coming to peace with it may be more difficult.

STEPS TOWARD RECONCILATION

Sue and Howard found RESOLVE support groups very helpful, as they worked their way through the infertility journey. Sue and Howard were struggling with the issue about when was the right time to stop treatment. Sue told me: "I remember being in our first support group, saying there has to be an end to this. So we always thought at some point we were going to stop. It won't necessarily be when we have a child. I think you should consider that as an equal option. Having a child is not necessarily the outcome for everybody. For some it is being childfree. People get understandably stuck on 'I am going to do this until I have my dream.' Their whole life gets completely drained away. I always looked at it as an equal option that I needed to understand. Is it for me?"

You also have to remember that, when you decide to end your treatment, it doesn't mean that your dreams of having a child be a part of your life has to end as well. There are always the options of adoption or surrogacy that are available to you. But you need to consider each of these as separate decisions. Each is one step in the many steps that we all face as we make choices about our lives and the lifestyles we choose to live. Adoption or surrogacy may or may not be the next steps for you.

In each case, it is important to make an informed decision based on all of the information you can get. You should consult with your doctors and any support staff involved with your treatment. Educate yourselves by reading and consulting with resources like RESOLVE. Talk with other people who have been through this decision to get additional insights and support to help you solidify your own thoughts and feelings. Spend a lot of time talking with your partner so you both understand each other's feelings about what the next step should be. You want to come to some mutual agreement in regards to this all-important decision. When you gather all of the information you can, using the resources I have mentioned, you can feel that your decision is based on as much knowledge as possible. With a clear understanding of your choices, you can plug in the pieces that feel right for you, and then make a decision that fits your particular circumstances.

I think making this decision is hardest when your doctors have not been able to pinpoint the reason for your infertility. Nobody goes into infertility treatment lightly. We are all hopeful that it will work. When we understand what the medical problem is that stops us from getting pregnant, then we usually have something tangible to work with in making these tough decisions. We know our treatment options and can pinpoint what kind of treatment might be successful. The doctors are better able to target specific treatment possibilities to our needs, and they are often able to measure when treatments are or are not successful through laboratory work and blood tests, or through other methods, such as ultrasounds. Through trials, testing, and examinations, our doctors can begin to better assess the likelihood of successful treatment in our individual cases. When we don't know what the cause of the infertility is, it feels like we are just shooting in the dark. There may always be that kernel of hope that, if I just try something else, then maybe I will be successful. It is hardest to take control and decide to stop under these circumstances. Again following the steps outlined above may prove useful to you, as you go through this process.

Howard talked about what worked best for them. "We were going by stages," he said. "We knew that when we did the egg donation that was our last try... My decisions were: what are we doing now. I know what lies ahead, but I don't want to think about it until I have to. We went to the "ABC's of Adoption" seminar at the same time we went to ones about living childfree. Then, I was just taking it one stage at a time."

Sue added: "We would go through one treatment, and then maybe we [would] need one more round of this for closure. It definitely evolved over time. Everybody has a different endurance level. We were really in sync for these steps along the way, and we would talk about: do we think we can do one more? It was more like a step-by-step thing."

Patricia Irwin Johnston writes in her book, *Taking Charge of Infertility*, about the painful issues involved when you are considering giving up treatment. She lists the following painful realizations:

- Even in having taken charge of your infertility you still could not control it. That hurts.
- Losing the dream of a jointly conceived child hurts.
- Losing genetic continuity hurts.
- Giving up on the desire to experience being or making pregnant hurts.
- Facing the idea of choosing an alternative route to parenthood hurts.(17)

TAKING TIME TO GRIEVE

You may find that you need to take some time off after you have made the decision to stop infertility treatment. Ms. Johnston talks about all of the hurt associated with making the decision to stop treatment. The emotion of grief goes hand in hand with the sense of hurt and loss you will feel. You may need time to work through this grief process before you move on to the next step, whatever that may be. You and your partner will need time to comfort each other and grieve in your own ways. Be aware that your grieving processes may be different, and you may need different lengths of time to work through this grief. You may have to give your partner some space and time alone to work through some of these feelings. Rushing won't help. It is critical that you continue to talk with each other or somebody else about what you are thinking and feeling, and that you allow your partner to express what he or she needs to work through this difficult time.

This may be another point where you want to seek help via a support group or an individual counselor. Sometimes it can help to just talk with friends or family members or others that may have experienced a similar turning point in their lives. Some people prefer to consult a spiritual advisor from their religion. There is no single answer. You may want to seek out a counselor who specializes in working with couples who have struggled with infertility issues. Their expertise can be invaluable. Sometimes making time and space, or taking a break, are necessary.

Taking a break may mean choosing to have a moratorium on making any further decisions about treatment or other options to achieve parenthood. You may not want to think about it for awhile and just give yourself time to emotionally recharge. Often, it is best to wait, and reflect later on what the next step might be. Also give yourself permission to change your mind. You and your partner do want to have some agreement on about how long your time-off period should be. It helps to know when you will take a look at the next step again, if there is going to be one. Give yourselves permission to re-evaluate this time-off as your needs dictate. I will look more specifically at the psychological issues associated with grief and loss in relation to infertility problems in Chapters 10 and 11.

In her book, *Taking Charge of Infertility*, Ms. Johnston does a wonderful job of detailing clues to help you recognize when it may be time for you to look at ending treatment. They include the following list:

- When either of you become more pessimistic than optimistic about the outcome of your treatment regimen.
- When one or the other of you comes to dread or resent the process of the treatment protocol.
- When any one of your resources—time, money, physical capacity, emotional energy—has reached a critical low that is affecting your ability to function well in your relationship with your partner.
- When your ability to function effectively with family and friends or in your job has been impaired.

• When any one of your resources—time, money, physical capacity, emotional energy—has reached a critical low that could impair your ability to successfully pursue a parenting option that you and your partner have already discussed as a positive alternative.

• When either of you finds that he or she has been spending more and more time thinking about one or more options other than treatment.(18)

You both may be thinking it is time to stop, but neither of you feels comfortable saying it out loud, for fear of upsetting your partner. Also, saying it out loud makes it begin to feel like a reality, when you haven't wanted to face up to this yet. The indicators outlined above are strong guidelines, and you should take them as potential signals to begin exploring this path. What Ms. Johnston is basically saying is that, when ongoing infertility treatment is impacting other significant areas of your life in very negative ways, you need to take a look at what you can do to inhibit that process.

Even if you decide to stop treatment, you still have two options for becoming parents. In the next two chapters, we will look at the areas of surrogacy and adoption. By using a surrogate, you may still be able to have a genetic link to your future child, which will not be true of adoption. Adoption, however, is a very common alternative that infertile couples pursue to hold onto their dream of having a child and being parents. Choosing to stop treatment does not necessarily mean you have to lose your dream of having a family. You may decide to live childfree, though, and this alternative is covered extensively in Chapter 10. The difficult decision to stop treatment is the first in a sequence of hard choices we face in the infertility journey. Many couples consider all these possibilities simultaneously, and find that one decision can help bring closure to another. It's good to consider all the alternatives, but sometimes, as Howard and Sue said, it's good to make decisions one step at a time. This can be the hardest part of the infertility journey.

CHAPTER 8
SURROGACY

We have heard the word surrogacy used in the media in recent years. Surrogacy is a type of collaborative reproduction used when a woman in unable to carry a child safely to full term. In this situation, a woman finds another woman who is willing to carry her child throughout the pregnancy. Surrogacy can involve using a woman's retrieved eggs, her husband's sperm, or both, it can also involve the use of a donated egg, sperm, or both, or a donated embryo. Surrogacy usually involves an IVF procedure, followed by embryo transfers to the surrogate.

A surrogate can be somebody you know, like a family member or a friend, or somebody else who is willing to volunteer to help carry a baby to full term. Recruited surrogates that you don't know are usually compensated, but they don't do this for the money. I have attended seminars where I heard women speak about why they wanted to be surrogates. Both in cases where they knew the person and did not, these women have spoken about their desire to help people have a child, who otherwise would not be able to have one. Their reasons are genuinely altruistic. Their willingness to offer this gift to somebody else is the ultimate act of kindness and selflessness. Surrogacy is one way that some infertile couples can still be the genetic parents of their children. Sometimes, only the father can become the genetic parent. Surrogacy also gives the couple an opportunity to support a pregnancy and follow the natural development of their child.

There are a number of things to consider if you find yourself thinking about surrogacy as a treatment option for yourself. Numerous questions arise in relation to this practice. First, you need to ask yourself whether you want to use somebody you know or not. If you do, you need to think about the nature of your relationship with this woman. How often do you see her? How will it impact your relationship to have her carry your child? Does she share the same belief system you do in terms of medical attention and prenatal care? What are her ideas about her healthcare during her pregnancy? What I mean by this is: are her beliefs around nutrition, exercise, and abstaining from drug or alcohol use the same as yours? How will her surrogacy impact your relationship after the child is born? What role will she be playing in your child's life after the child is born? These critical issues need to be looked at carefully and discussed at length with your surrogate.

If your surrogate has a significant-other, all these issues should also be discussed with that person before you pursue this type of arrangement. Your surrogate's partner will be with her on an ongoing basis throughout the pregnancy and will play a part in helping her through her pregnancy. If the significant-other shares your beliefs, that person can lend support to all of you throughout the pregnancy. If that person has different values regarding the pregnancy, it can cause stress for you and your surrogate, and this can have an impact on how the pregnancy goes.

LEGAL CONSIDERATIONS

Whether you use somebody you know well or somebody you don't know, there are many things that need to be spelled out in writing in some type of legal arrangement. You should definitely consult an attorney who specializes in infertility treatment if you choose this path. Legally speaking, surrogacy is the most risky form of infertility treatment, since the surrogate is actually the one who gives birth to the child. In Chapter 6, we looked at a lot of the legal issues involved with infertility treatment, and made reference to the complexities associated with surrogacy. The laws associated with surrogacy are constantly changing, and can vary considerably from state to state. Some states are more lenient or strict than others. For example, as recently as last year, surrogacy was not legal in Indiana.

Some of the specifics you need to spell out in a contract include: who will pay the medical expenses, and how medical costs will be paid. The contract should be clear about whose insurance will cover the medical costs. Will your surrogate be compensated? Will her compensation vary, depending on her complications in pregnancy? What if the surrogate mother needs to stop working, because of pregnancy-related problems? The contract needs to outline how she should be compensated for her time off of work. What should happen if there is a problem with the pregnancy? The contract needs to address the issue of who would determine what medical treatment should be provided for the baby and mother. Think about the process that will allow these decisions to be made. Your doctor and her doctor may be different, and you may want to have an arrangement where they consult together about any problems during the pregnancy. What will that process entail? There are many contingencies that could arise in the course of your surrogate's pregnancy, and your legal arrangement should address them thoroughly. Using an experienced lawyer is highly recommended.

Postnatal questions should also be addressed. For example, you might want to think about is how the baby will be fed. If you want the baby to be breastfed, you need to work out an arrangement with the surrogate mother. You and your family and the surrogate will need to reach an understanding about what information you will give your child about how she or he was born. You must be consistent regarding the messages you give. We will be discussing disclosure in greater detail in Chapter 17. Surrogacy agreements usually spell out future disclosure limitations, if there are to be any. Visitation expectations, if any, are also usually included in these agreements, and these can range from complete future anonymity to regular, frequent contact.

A VERY SPECIAL SITUATION

Surrogacy is a fairly rare practice, and there may be no one you know and can talk with, who has had personal experience with this situation. I believe it is a good idea to talk with people who have gone through this complicated process. If you want to get more information regarding surrogacy, you can contact RESOLVE, and they can put you in touch with other people who have used this procedure. They also hold seminars where all aspects of surrogacy are discussed. There is also a group called the Organization of Parents through Surrogacy, which is a good place to get resource information. Finally, there is an organization called the American Surrogacy Center. You can find out more information about these programs in Chapter 22.

Because surrogacy is such a special situation, I believe it is important to have all parties involved see a counselor whenever the potential use of surrogacy is being considered. Many clinics are now making this a requirement. It is preferable that this counselor be somebody who specializes in the area of infertility treatment, since he or she will be familiar with the unique issues that may arise when choosing this form of infertility treatment. Your counselor's knowledge and experience can help prepare you—and, in fact, empower you—so you will be able to face the issues that may arise in the future. This is particularly critical if you are using a surrogate who you do not know.

It is becoming a standard practice for people who agree to be donors or surrogates to undergo a complete battery of psychological tests. Understanding the surrogate's psychological makeup is invaluable in trying to determine if she is the best possible candidate for this type of procedure. It also gives you additional insights and understanding of the motivating reasons for her willingness to participate in a surrogate arrangement. Believe it or not, there are some people that will volunteer to do this for financial reasons. You want to try to be as certain as possible that the person who is agreeing to be your surrogate has no history of drug or alcohol abuse, since this can directly impact the fetus. You also want to try to be aware of any potential psychological history or current problems that might impact the success of the pregnancy. Even women with perfect mental health can find giving up a baby they carry for nine months psychologically trying.

There are many people today who view surrogacy with skeptical, and sometimes critical, eyes. Members of our society still impose their opinions on people who choose surrogacy. Sometimes, this is based on their own personal, religious, or moral belief systems. People may have a hard time understanding why you would choose to have somebody else carry your child. Your surrogate may also face the stigmas and judgments of others. The media is picking up these stories on a more consistent basis. We have heard stories about a mother carrying her daughter's child and siblings being surrogates. When my sister found out that we were having infertility problems, she offered to be a surrogate for us. Surrogacy requires courage and a high level of commitment by all those involved.

Once again, the critical piece for you is to explore your heart and your innermost thoughts and feelings. You will need to determine the comfort level you and your partner have with the idea of surrogacy. You will need to find a surrogate who can match your needs and desires. Then, before you proceed, you will need to ask yourselves about how family and close friends would react to this type of arrangement? Disclosure becomes a huge issue with surrogacy. How and when would you disclose your pursuit of surrogacy to your family, your friends and, most critically, to your child? These are issues that should be resolved in advance, and everyone involved should agree and be at peace with the arrangement.

This is another reason it is helpful to see some type of counselor. They can help guide you through these questions and come to the conclusions that feel right for you. They can also be available to you after your child is born, and help you address the issues that may arise as your child begins to grow. In surrogacy, there can be issues around bonding for you and your spouse and the surrogate after the child is born. These issues often need to be worked through with the help of a skilled professional. It is wise to lay the groundwork for this in advance by initiating a relationship with a counselor, who can help you through this potentially challenging course of postnatal adjustments.

It should be clear from what we have discussed so far that the whole area of infertility treatment raises a wide range of psychological issues that need to be closely examined. This is the focus of Chapter 11 and, before you decided to pursue surrogacy, you should read this chapter. Alternatives to surrogacy include adoption and deciding to live childfree, which are covered in the next two chapters. Choosing surrogacy has not been that common in the past, but advancements in reproductive technology are making it more readily available to more couples. Ongoing scientific advancements may make the possibility of pursuing this option more attractive to couples, especially those who have a strong desire for genetically related children.

Surrogacy is challenging—it stretches our cultural boundaries around parenthood. But more and more people are choosing to push this social envelope, because they feel it is right for them. Making this choice is another way that some people become proactive and assertive in their pursuit of a family. Many surrogates, in fact, feel that they are empowering the future parents and the child that they carry. Surrogates often feel that they get to give greatest gift that can be given. As long as there are women with the courage to be surrogates, there will be couples willing to accept this profound gift of life and a future family.

CHAPTER 9
ADOPTION CONSIDERATIONS

The roller coaster ride of infertility typically takes us through a period of treatment first. Often, it's not until these medical alternatives fail that we begin to look at other options. Most couples consider the idea of adopting a child early on, but many don't give this alternative serious consideration until their infertility treatment fails. Some people have very low odds of succeeding through treatment, and a lot of time and money can be spent pursuing a possibility that never materializes. Adoption takes time, too, but it is the one alternative that guarantees you will get a child and become a family in the end. Adoption has certainty, and this has appeal for many infertile couples.

Sue and Howard, the couple who chose an egg donor option, spoke to me about going to adoption information seminars. They did this while they were still in the midst of pursuing IVF treatments, just so they would have information about all of their options. Howard told me: "We went to the ABC's of Adoption seminar, and all these things about adoption, at the same time we went to ones about living childfree."

It can be difficult to switch gears and go from doing everything you can to have a biological or genetic child to seriously examining the area of adoption. This is not necessarily something you want to do overnight, but giving adoption consideration during your treatment process can be a good thing. Adoption may be something you never would have considered in the past. You and your partner (or you as a future single parent) want to give it a lot of thought. The most significant question you must explore within yourself is whether you believe you are capable of adopting? Will you be able to love, accept, and bond with a child who has no genetic or biologic link with you? The flip side of this is: will this child ultimately be able to love and bond with you?

Patricia Irwin Johnston addresses this paramount question of adoption, and uses it to explore whether adoption is for you or not. She describes the people who are ready for adoption saying: "They understand that in adoption their loss of control may, for a time, be magnified as they give over control to an adoption intermediary or cast their lot to young birthparents to choose them. They allow themselves to feel some anger about this and then to accept it as a necessary loss. They recognize that they will not have a genetic connection to their child and will not continue their family bloodlines. But, over what for many is a significant amount of time, they come to feel that in parenting a child by adoption they will extend themselves and their family into the future in profound social and emotional ways. While they will lose the opportunity to create a child conceived by the blending of their own genes with those of their much loved partner, they are pleased that the two of them will parent together, and they like the equal footing that adoption allows them as parents. They have thought about the two losses—emotional and physical—attached to the expectations they had about the pregnancy and birth experience and have come to believe that the nine months of pregnancy is not particularly significant compared to a lifetime of active parenting."(19)

Kate and Eric and I spoke at length about their experience with adoption. They agreed with Ms. Johnston's descriptions of adoption. They described some of the ups and downs they encountered on their path to do an international adoption in China of their daughter, Leah. Eric, in particular, addressed the loss of control issues described in the previous quote. He said, "For me, and other people like me, you have to figure out how much demeaning treatment you can take. Like once you get into this, you know you are going to be looked at. You are going to be fingerprinted. You are going to have the FBI look at you. You are going to have to be licensed by the state as a licensed foster parent in the state of Illinois. That's just the baseline. That is something nobody can avoid no matter what they do. Our agency prepared us well for that. On top of that, how much can you take from the system? You have to sort of swallow that. Then you have a whole lot of choices and you have to figure out which one is palatable to you. Once you get past that first phase, you then have to wait in line. [It took] a long time to learn that the program we were in was probably going to take us."

Kate reinforced the strong positive aspects of being an adoptive parent that Ms. Johnston described. Kate told me, "I didn't want to wait around for a birth mother to choose me....The most amazing thing is how secure it feels to be an adoptive parent. I never thought it would feel that way. How less narcissistic [it is] that your child is not your genetics... You can't blame it on that. Certain traits get picked up regardless of genetics. People say to me: 'She sounds just like you and looks just like you.'" Then they both laughed, because Kate and Eric are caucasian.

When I asked Eric about how others reacted to his adopting a child, Eric told me: "One reaction I have gotten—from some adults who have found out I have adopted—is they start praising me for how selfless I must be. I didn't adopt for selfless reasons. I wanted a family. Maybe you could call it selfish reasons, or at least no more selfless than any other parent...There could be more than one motive to adopt, more than one mindset where you find yourselves in the adoptive parent category. We always turn to people who say she is so lucky—we turn to them and say, "'No we are the lucky ones,' because she is so great." Kate nodded her head in approval and smiled.

There will be ups and downs no matter what method you pursue to try and become a parent. When we were going through our infertility treatment, we had chosen a woman to be our donor, and we were all set to go, when we found out she got pregnant. We had to start from square one all over again. It was terribly frustrating and disappointing. This experience is very similar to that of an adopting couple working with a birth mother who changes her mind, and decides not to give her baby up for adoption. While adoption is the one alternative that will eventually make you parents, that certainty doesn't mean there won't be ups and downs. Problems can, and likely will, arise. Be aware of that. Go into these situations with your eyes open, and expect a roller coaster ride. Then, you won't be as immobilized when the unexpected happens.

APPROACHES TO ADOPTION

When you are looking into adoption there are many important decisions that you need to make. One of the first things you need to think about is whether you want to do an adoption through an agency or go through a lawyer to arrange a private adoption? Do you think you would consider an international adoption?

Mark McDermott, JD, a legal expert, takes a look at what the legal differences are in these cases in an article for *Family Building* magazine. He points out that: "From a legal point of view, every case must be either an agency adoption or an independent (non agency) adoption. What makes a case one or the other is the way in which the parental rights pass from the birth parents to the adoptive parents. In an agency case, there are two steps. First, the birth parents rights are relinquished to an agency. Second, the agency consents to an adoption by a particular adoptive parent or parents. In an independent adoption, there is only one step. The birth parents give consent directly to a particular adoptive parent or parents."(20)

Do you think you might consider an international adoption? If you would, there are some specifics that Mr. McDermott thinks are critical for you to know. He says: "When children born in another country are adopted by US citizens, the controlling law is the law of the child's country of origin. The adoptive parent's final decree of adoption will be granted by the court or other authority in the child's country of birth. A few countries do confer legal authority on the adoptive parents to finalize the adoption in the adoptive parent's country. In either of these scenarios, the action by the foreign country, which results in making the adoptive parents the legal parents of the child, does not automatically make the child a U.S. citizen. Consequently, a visa must be obtained for the child to enter the United States. Previously, it was necessary for children adopted from other countries to go through the naturalization process to become U.S. citizens. A February 27, 2001 law made citizenship automatic in most cases when the child enters the United States as a permanent resident."(21) Be sure you check with a lawyer to see what laws are relevant to your specific situation, including current immigration law.

Once you make the decision to adopt, there are numerous questions you need to carefully consider. You need to determine if you will be doing the adoption yourself, perhaps with a lawyer, or whether you will choose to work through an adoption agency. Another part of this question is whether you want to adopt a child who shares your ethnic background or would you consider adopting a child from a different ethnic or racial background? You also want to ask yourself what age do you want this child to be? Are you tied to the idea of having a brand new baby? Are you willing to think about adopting a child who may be older? Would you consider adopting more than one child, for example a child and a sibling? Do you want an open adoption, where the birth parent would possibly have an ongoing involvement with the child, or a closed or confidential adoption? What will you tell family and friends about the adoption? What will you tell your adopted child about where he or she came from? Answers to these all important questions will help dictate what your next steps will be.

Pat Johnston identifies the resources you need to examine and explore to help you determine the right type of adoption for you. She suggests you think about four specific areas, and writes:

> Time may be a pressing issue. The wait for a healthy white newborn through an agency can be up to ten years in some parts of the country. This leads some couples to explore non-agency adoption, or non-infant adoption, or trans-racial or international adoption, or adopting a child with some special health or emotional needs. Your own advancing age may influence the options open to you in adoption.
>
> Money may be a factor. Some agencies assess adopters a flat fee and some charge using a sliding scale. Some independent adoptions can involve relatively minimal legal costs and modest medical expenses not covered by a birthparent's insurance and others can involve living expenses, psychological counseling, legal advice in two states, travel, etc. The same is true with international adoptions.
>
> Emotional reserves may lead some couples to decide that they want the 'protection' afforded by a traditional, confidential agency adoption, while others are interested in risking some emotional pain in order to have more control or save time, etc.
>
> Your physical resources may influence the age and the relative health and the number of children you are prepared to parent at once.(22)

In Kate and Eric's case, time was an issue because they began the adoption process in their forties. They also felt strongly they wanted to go through an established adoption agency. They did not want to wait a long time for a child, and they were not tied to the idea of getting a brand new baby. This steered them on the course of an international adoption. I asked them to talk about how they chose going to China and what things they considered in looking at an international adoption. I thought Eric had some valuable information to offer. He said: "I compared all of the different programs, all of the different countries, and what we had to do to satisfy their requirements, including domestic. With a domestic adoption you almost have to audition for the birth mother, who then chooses you. Some countries you have to go down twice. Of course, with all of these countries the rules change from moment to moment, as different government administrator's move out of their jobs, and different regimes and laws get passed. But at that time, China's program seemed the best to me. It seemed straightforward, sensible—all of the requirements seemed realistic. They did a background check, criminal, and a social worker checked you out. But it seemed like they were very objective. If you meet these requirements, then you get on the list, and you were selected."

Kate added: "There was another big factor for me. Some of the Latin countries had issues about whether the children are surrendered and whether mothers did it voluntarily. I am sure there are those who do that, but I felt there was a fear that a mother would be talked into it because of the money. There is a lot of money coming into these countries from the adoption market."

Whether you choose an international or a domestic adoption, there are similarities in some ways. In both cases you will still have to undergo a home study program. Reliable agencies will require you to take classes and will have you undergo the intense scrutiny described above. Kate referred to it as "the agencies being cops for the kids." She felt this "was a good thing." There will be some kind of waiting period involved. That will depend on the place you get the child, the ethnicity or race, and the age of the child. There are wonderful programs and resources available throughout the United States to help you with this transition.

Kate and Eric, for example, found a doctor who specialized in working with Chinese babies. This doctor was able to give them lots of valuable information about what potential medical problems to look for in the baby. There are certain common things doctors see in kids adopted from China, such as vitamin deficiencies, so their doctor sent them with vitamins and a wealth of knowledge when they went to China. They also linked up with a program composed of other families who have adopted kids from China. They did this so they would have a support network in place and know other people with kids who shared Leah's cultural heritage. The state of Illinois offered a program where a child from China could get free physical or speech therapy, if needed, once they were brought here. There may be similar programs in your area, depending on funding and where your child is adopted. When you do a domestic adoption through an agency, there should be a social worker available to offer you guidance and link you with the appropriate support network once your adoption is completed.

Today, there is even a medical specialty called "adoption medicine." It has been created to accommodate the needs of the increasing number of Americans who are choosing international adoptions. These doctors will evaluate and review medical records of prospective adopted children from different countries. They will also do post-adoption consultations. Kids from other countries may have a higher number of infections and ailments, such as tuberculosis, or medical problems associated with poor diet. An increasing number of physicians are available to offer pre-adoption counseling, and they have specific knowledge about medical issues that may be associated with adopting a child from a specific country. They can often be proactive in their medical treatment for these adopted kids. For example, they might recommend a specific vitamin supplement because they know that the diet of a specific country does not have this vitamin available.

Whether you choose a domestic or international adoption, you should find out what medical and background information you can get on the child. If you can get information on their family's psychological and drug or alcohol history, that would be very useful information as well. Get as complete and accurate a medical history as possible. This can be difficult with kids from other countries. Kate and Eric told me that at the orphanage where they got their daughter, the kids were left with notes pinned in their pockets to provide information about the child. Some children were left without any note at all! So information about their medical history—or even the age of the child—may not exist, or when it does, it may not be exact or accurate. You want to make sure the child you receive has a thorough medical exam with somebody reliable, and this should be done as quickly as possible.

You will also need to get all the information you can about what travel costs will be, particularly if you do an international adoption. There may be requirements about how long you need to stay before and after the adoption. You should find out what accommodations are available for you, and what the costs for this would be over the expected time period. You should find out if there will be any additional expenses associated with paperwork in the other country. If you have other children already, you should find out if you will be allowed to bring your other children with you. You should decide whether you would do this, or think about what arrangements you could make for your other children, if you didn't bring them. International adoption can be both time-consuming and unpredictable, leading sometimes to unplanned delays. Gather as much information as you possibly can about the logistics of executing your adoption.

Be sure and talk with others who have used the agency you selected, if you do choose an agency adoption. Talk with them about what their experiences were in the country you have selected. Find out how things went after they returned to this country. Get feedback both in terms of the health of the child and in terms of any glitches they experienced in the paperwork or other legal issues. If you decide to use an attorney, make sure you get somebody who has expertise in this area, and again try to talk with others who have worked with this lawyer. As prospective adoptive parents, you need to be as informed as you can be regarding the issues outlined above.

TRANSRACIAL ADOPTIONS

If you choose to adopt a child who is of a different race, or multiracial, or of a different ethnicity, then you should think about how this will impact your lives. You and your child may encounter prejudice. If you are adopting a child with a partner, you need to discuss these issues openly and frankly to ensure you understand your comfort level with this potential dilemma. Imagine how coming face-to-face with this potential prejudice might impact your child and how you might handle it. Thinking these issues through and considering how you might handle them is a means to prepare and empower yourself as you go through this process. You have to define for yourselves how large a role it will play in your adoption process. These are all questions to be explored.

Michelle Hughes, a woman with experience in the area of transracial adoptions, addresses this particular area in a 2002 issue of *Hope* magazine. She gives excellent recommendations to potential parents who are considering adopting kids across racial lines. She provides a mental checklist of questions to ask yourself to see if this is the right path for you. She starts by saying that these parents "require an education in adoption plus race." She tells potential adoptive parents to consider the following:

- Take an honest look at your true feeling as an individual and as a couple about race. Do you consciously or subconsciously differentiate people based on race? (Hint: Most of us do, as it is a taught behavior in this country; however, taught behaviors can be changed.)
- Are you willing to communicate about race? You will need to have frank discussions with your child on this subject. In addition, you will probably need to have frank discussions with family, friends and the public on race.
- Are you willing to incorporate another racial culture in your life? Remember that it is not the child's sole job to assimilate into your culture but the family's responsibility to incorporate and celebrate different racial cultures within your individual family structure.
- Are you aware of racism, both in its overt and subtle forms in this country? Will you be willing to be empathetic to your child's experiences with racism? Will you be ready to deal

with your own new experiences with racism? (Hint: You have to be able to recognize them in order to address them.) Will you search out the tools to help your child cope with racism so they become people with healthy self identities? Are you willing to help eradicate racism?

• Do you have diverse friendships (not just associations) now? If not, why not? Are you willing to change that? Diverse friendships will serve both as resources and role models for you and your children.

• Are you willing to deal with the unique challenges of being a multiracial family? Being a multiracial family is very conspicuous, and complete privacy does not exist. Consider how will you handle being stared at, becoming an unofficial spokesperson for adoption, and listening to rude questions and comments?

• Are you willing to relish the benefits of being a multiracial family, including meeting new people, making new friends, and learning new cultures?(23)

In my discussion with Kate and Eric, I asked them about how they would address the cultural issues with their daughter, Leah. Eric told me: "We tell her as much as we know. We were in China trying to find out and anticipate what she would ask. We came away and tried to ask the questions she would. Some people are really into it and get a teacher to teach them Chinese. We do more with families with children from China."

Kate told me, "Richard has taken on the obligation and the responsibility of marching with Leah in the Chinese New Year's parade every year."

OPEN OR CLOSED ADOPTIONS

When looking at the decision of an open versus a closed (or confidential) adoption, there are a few things to think about. This is another place where you have real choice and can feel you are taking some control. You will need to choose which type of adoption you want. Be clear with the agency or independent person or attorney that is assisting you about the direction you choose to go. Make sure that this is a style of adoption that they practice. Some agencies agree with the philosophy of open adoptions, some do not.

There are lots of different levels of openness in adoptions. You can decide how much contact you and your child will have with the birth parent and their family. What will be the nature of the contact? It can be in person, by telephone, and in writing. In making this choice, you must be certain that you will feel comfortable spending time with the birth family and having them as an ongoing part of your child's life. In your discussions, be sure you come to a clear understanding about who the child will see and how often this will occur. Any agreements that you make should be put in writing, and using an attorney or intermediary would be a good idea. You should spell things out in the most appropriate legal way. Keep in mind that your feelings may change as time goes on. Sometimes, the birth parents feelings change as well.

This happened with a friend of mine, who had done an open adoption with the birth mother. They adopted a new baby directly from the birth mother with the help of an adoption agency. Initially the birth mother wanted to be involved and see the child every month or two. But as time went on, her interest and involvement waned, and she wouldn't show up for appointed visits. It is critical to consider the impact on the child of the specific arrangements that are made. It can be very confusing for them, if people step in and out of their lives. There needs to be some consistency in the message they are given in this regard. Also, remember the way your child views adoptions will change with time and will be influenced by your perceptions and the messages you give them. This is true for and the birth parents, too, if they continue to be involved in the child's life.

Closed adoptions have been the norm for a very long time, and most adoptions are still closed. The laws related to adoption records vary from state to state, and many adopted children can get access to their records as adults today. Most adopted children do not have contact with the birth parent and their family while they are growing up, but an increasing number of adult adopted children are seeking out their families of origin. My husband has four adopted sisters, and they have all sought out their families of origin at one time or another in their lives. This is part of a general trend toward greater openness in adoption. This trend can be seen in the ongoing changes in the law around adoption records, and the ever-increasing number of open adoptions.

There is no right or wrong answer about having an open or closed adoption. Some people go so far as to never tell their child they are adopted. When this happens, there is always the risk that the child will find out later, and live this experience traumatically. Sometimes, it is the birth mother who wants privacy, and she will dictate how open or closed the adoption becomes. There is a wide spectrum of possible arrangements, and you may be uncertain yourself how open or closed you would want your own adoption to be. Each circumstance is different, as is each child, and you should give careful thought to your philosophy and make sure that your partner agrees. Ultimately, circumstances may dictate what you can do, but always keep in mind the best interests of your child. This includes thinking about what they might want to know in the future. The challenge of parenting is to let your child flourish and become who they are, so think carefully about your child's potential future issues with identity. You will likely need to decide for them whether having an open or closed adoption will better help them achieve a healthy self-knowledge.

THE BONDING CHALLENGE

Many people have specific notions about the age of the child they want to adopt. Often, this is driven by a desire to have a baby, in order to have the full child-parent bonding experience from the earliest age. Of course we all know that demand for newborn babies is high, and they are available in fewer numbers. You must be prepared to wait a longer time, if adopting a newborn is what you choose to do. Some people prefer not to have to deal with all things that go along with having a newborn child, such as sleeplessness, changing diapers, and multiple feedings. Couples experiencing secondary infertility sometimes chose to adopt older children, so their adopted children will be closer in age to their own children and more quickly integrated into their families. Other people feel that older kids have a greater need for a home, and adopting them provides an immediate opportunity to parent in a profound and transformative way. Different people bring different attitudes to adoption and the decision about age. Think about the aspects of parenting that you feel will help build a stronger bond between you and your adoptive child, and use this as one of your guides.

There are many research studies that present assorted opinions about how and when a child's personality is shaped. Some believe it begins with genetics where personality traits are carried and passed on. Some believe a child's personality is basically constructed by the time they are two years old. Other people believe that the environment and people that children are raised with can have an ongoing impact on their personality, growth, and development. Sorting all of these ideas out may seem complex, and researchers have found this question too complicated to resolve. There's probably a lot of truth in each one these ideas. You should think about this question, and come to terms with your own understanding and beliefs. This will influence your philosophy about adoption, and help you decide how you and your adopted child will fit into your world and the world around you. Understanding your beliefs and acting on them will likely go a long way towards making this a successful transition.

Adoption is a challenging process, and the most critical part of the challenge is bonding with your adoptive child. Even if you go into adoption with the best of intentions, it can initially be hard to build a bond with a child or baby who feels like a stranger. This new child has no biological link to you, may not share your ethnicity, race, or any of your physical characteristics. When you do decide to adopt a child, it can really challenge your commitment as a parent, and your commitment to each other as a couple. As a couple you need to talk extensively prior to the adoption about why you want to adopt and what the adoption will mean to you. You both need to have a similar passion about your desire to have this new child become the new center of your world. Spend time considering your "world view" in terms of the development of a child. Ask yourself if this new child needs to fit into this world view, or will you give this child permission to alter your personal perspectives? What things can you do as a parent that will directly impact the development of your child? What messages do you want to convey to your child about the world around him and how he fits into that world? What messages do you want to convey about how this child will fit into your life and culture?

Your commitment as individuals and as a couple to be both physically and emotionally available to your adoptive child must be strong. This new child will unyieldingly demand that he or she becomes the priority in your life. Your acceptance, ability and willingness to put other important areas of your life (like your career) into a less prominent position are key elements in the success of your bonding process. Ask yourself how willing you really are to make these adjustments in your thinking and your life? Does your partner have a similar perspective on these priorities?

Children of different ages will bond in different ways. If you adopt a child who is not a newborn, the bonding process has different elements. The older the child, the more of a chance the child has had to develop personality traits and behavioral patterns. You will have to overcome that child's previous experiences in significant relationships, and it is probable that many of those experiences will have been negative, since this child has been put up for adoption. At the same time, you can never change what your child has encountered in the past. There will be lots of issues around trust with an older child. This child will want and need ongoing proof from you, that you will be able and willing to care for and care about them.

There will likely be lots of initial testing from an older child. They will likely challenge you to continue to demonstrate your desire to love them and make them a real member of your family. Angry outbursts and temper tantrums are examples of testing. Some children may cling to you and not want you out of their sight. They need to know that you are there all of the time. If you give your attention to somebody else, the child may engage in a behavior that will attract your attention again. This includes negative and positive behaviors. These initial weeks and months will set the stage for developing relationships that you will be building on in the years to come.

For new adoptive parents this can be a very trying and difficult time. It can also be a rewarding time, as your child begins to respond to the love, support, home, family, and structure you bring into his or her life. Structure is something many of these children may not have had before. Something as simple as eating three meals a day, at the same time every day, may be a new experience for some of these children. They may have come from a place where food was at a premium, and they were not sure where—and if—the next meal was coming. Hoarding food and toys is not unusual behavior for some of these children. The child will need reassurance that you will not repeat the previous patterns of abandonment.

Watching and facilitating the growth of these children can be incredibly rewarding and satisfying. It will require time and patience on everybody's part. You and your partner need to agree about how you will approach these types of problems, and you must both be consistent in your response to these displays of behavior. For those of you that adopt children from another culture who speak a different language, this will be an additional barrier that you will need to overcome. Facial expressions, gesturing, and consistent use of words and patterns of communication by you and your partner will enhance this process of transition for your child. Children are very adept at reading our faces, and they are extremely sensitive and intuitive to our emotions. It doesn't matter if they speak the same language or not. They pick up on the signals we send them, whether we are aware of it or not. Be aware of the messages you are sending to your adoptive child on these many levels.

For those who adopt newborns and babies, bonding issues may seem more easily resolved, but this is not necessarily the case. Even natural parents can have bonding issues, particularly with a difficult baby. Caring for a newborn is highly demanding, and takes over life. It's a twenty-four hour commitment from the very first moment without an end in sight. The challenge of parenting a newborn can snowball because of sleeplessness and the relentless demands for care. Adopting an older baby has its own challenges. Babies develop quickly, and much of their early development depends upon their interaction with a primary caregiver. A change of caregiver can be traumatic for a baby, and depending on their stage of development, the adjustment period can be stormy and difficult. The good news is that babies are generally quite responsive and adaptable, but as a new adoptive parent you will need to match their needs, which can be very challenging initially. Adopted babies are just as demanding as older adopted children, if in different ways. Rising to their needs is the key to good child-parent bonding.

If you adopt a baby, you will have to make disclosure decisions. Whatever decision you make, you should write this down, along with your reasons for deciding to do it this way. If your child ever discovers or wants to know about their origins, having the answer in writing may be invaluable to them. Some parents even write it as a letter to the child. Disclosure in this case is much like the disclosure issues associated with assisted reproduction that are explored in Chapter 17. Remember, you may not be around when your child wants to explore their origins, and putting what you know in writing can be a great gift to them. It can also serve you later in life by renewing your understanding of how the journey began for you.

Adoption is not easy. You will likely have to deal with acceptance issues in your larger family and in society generally. You will need to be ready to deal with these reactions and how they impact you and your child over time. Bonding is the key to good parenting, and adoption brings special challenges to this process. Your adopted child will need to discover who they are, and one part of this self-discovery may be a desire to explore their origins. This isn't always easy for an adoptive parent, but it is a natural part of an adopted child's search for self-understanding. Parenting is challenging and transformative, and that is one of the reasons so many of us pursue it so fervently. Being an adoptive parent is no less challenging and enriching for us and our children, and it is something you can choose to do. It is not a question of odds or probabilities or chance. This is the one option in the infertility journey where you have real choice, and you can decide, "Yes, I will be a parent."

CHAPTER 10
MAKING THE CHOICE TO LIVE CHILDFREE

When people go through infertility treatment it seems unfathomable to even think that they could one day make the choice to have no children. Treatment isn't easy, though, and sometimes it has only a small chance of success. Choosing to become parents through surrogacy or adoption remain options, but many people make the choice not to pursue these routes to parenthood for a variety of reasons. Some people feel strongly that if they cannot have a genetic link to their child their bonding won't be complete, and so they choose not to take the adoption road. Some people may not feel comfortable with the surrogacy option and the legal, psychological, and logistical complexities that are associated with this treatment choice.

There are a lot of losses associated with the decision to leave your dream of having children behind. These losses include the inability to carry on your "family line," the disappointment of never becoming a parent, and the loss of all the dreams you associated with that envisioned life. The loss of a genetic link to the future is a huge one for many people. When we begin our journey down the road of infertility treatment, nobody can really prepare us for how all-consuming it becomes. We all go into it with the hope and dream that we will be successful and be able to have a child. We cannot begin to predict the path our emotions will take us on as we make this journey. We have already looked at the lengths people will go to make this dream a reality. We make many sacrifices in all areas of our lives to achieve this precious goal.

Stopping treatment can trigger feelings of loss, as I described in a previous chapter. Making the decision to live childfree often triggers additional feelings of grief and mourning that can compound this previous sense of loss at stopping treatment. Grief and mourning are normal parts of the process people go through, when they stop treatment and begin moving toward the next possibility of living childfree. Deciding to live childfree is a distinctly different choice than the decision to stop treatment. When you choose to stop treatment, the dream of having a child can still remain alive through the possibilities of surrogacy or adoption. The decision to remain childfree, however, puts that desire to be a parent and have a family to rest forever.

PROCESSES OF MOURNING

In her 2002 article, "Mourning the Losses of Infertility," in *Family Building* magazine, Kim Kluger-Bell touches on some of the important focus areas for coming to terms with the end of treatment, the possibility of living childfree, and the losses associated with infertility. She describes the six-year struggle she and her husband went through, with failed IVF tries, failed egg donor attempts, and ectopic pregnancies. One of the things she wrote about was the importance of rituals, when a decision is made not to pursue treatment any further. For her and her husband this meant going to a beautiful serene place. They had decided to do a ceremony to help cope with the failed attempts, to say good bye to their unborn children, and to prepare themselves to move on.

She described their ritual as follows: "First, we lit a fire on the beach and burned all of the medical bills we had accumulated over the years we battled infertility. Then, we read each other the letters we had written to the children we had wanted and would never have. My husband threw a tiny silver box containing our letters into the sea. Then a most amazing thing happened. The gentle curve of a gray whale rose before us, not a hundred yards from where we stood."(24)

This was something they had decided to do together. It was a way for each of them to mourn individually, and together, for that future they dreamed about and now could admit was not going to happen. The distinction she makes between grief and mourning is a critical one and she goes on to define the difference. Mourning is really a description of the process, rituals and things we do to help ourselves cope with, and work through, our losses and grief. She goes on to specifically address mourning in relation to infertility. She states: "This is much more complicated when you are coping with the more intangible and on-going losses of infertility. Not only is there no actual person to mourn, but until you get to the point of deciding not to pursue another pregnancy you can't have any real closure on your losses. It's like waiting for a loved one to return home. After a long period of time your hopes begin to fade but you don't want to believe that they are gone for good. You can't fully grieve for them until you have arrived at the point of accepting that they will never return. This can leave you in a state of suspended animation or 'stuckness' for a very long period of time."(25)

You should be aware that there will be a lot of ups and downs as this process of grieving occurs. Eventually the downs will shorten in intensity and duration. There is no rule-of-thumb about how long this process will last. It differs for each individual. Ms. Kluger-Bell gives some very useful ideas on how to grieve the losses infertility produces, and if you follow these "tips" it will help you begin to move on and determine what the next step will be for you. Here are her tips on *Grieving the Losses of Infertility*:

- *Acknowledge the reality of your losses.* It is easy to underestimate the extent of your losses when you are dealing with infertility. Make a list of what you have been through: How many months and/or years have you spent trying to get pregnant? How many procedures have you been through? How much money have you spent? How many pregnancy losses have you experienced?

- *Let yourself have your feelings.* If you feel sad, let yourself be sad. If you're angry, be angry. If you feel intense jealousy, so be it. You won't feel any of these things forever. It is much better to have some compassion for yourself than to put yourself down for having these kinds of feelings.

- *Recognize that you cannot change the past, and that you have done nothing to deserve your infertility.* A lot of people blame themselves for having waited too long to start a family, or for having had previous pregnancies that they chose to terminate. Hindsight, as we all know, is always perfect. And remember bad things can happen to very good people.

- *Give yourself time to recover after major disappointments or when you're feeling depleted.* It's easy to lose track of how worn out you are after a long struggle with infertility. Be gentle with yourself. Take a break. Do things that make you feel refreshed and renewed.

• *Accept the fact that your struggle cannot go on forever and that there may come a time when you have to let go and move on.* It may be helpful to do something that signifies the end of your attempts to have a successful pregnancy—such as holding a ceremony, writing a letter, or going on a long awaited trip. Some people find comfort in announcing this ending to friends and family members in a letter that also lets them know how they can be most helpful at this time.(26)

You may find that it is difficult for you to do any or all of the things on this list. See what feels right for you. You may not be able to do some of these things now, but you may find later that they feel more comfortable as time passes on. Be aware of these options, and keep them on hand as a useful tool, while you continue this process.

THE STRUGGLE FOR A NEW BEGINNING

In the midst our grief, the prospect of our future can seem bleak and empty. What do we want for our lives now? Without children and a family, what will we aspire to do or be? During mourning, it can seem difficult to reorient to a new beginning. Yet, if we think about it, there are many people who have decided not to have children be a part of their lives. Some of them have always known that they wanted to live their lives without children. There are others who always assumed they might have children, but came to realize later in life that they won't do it. Why do they make this choice? What enables them to make it, and what does it enable them to do in their lives?

There are a host of reasons that people make the decision not to have children. Some never meet a person they want to share this responsibility with, and they don't feel they want to bring up a child as a single parent. Some feel having no children offers them freedom that they enjoy. Others don't believe they would make good parents, or don't want the financial or emotional obligations this commitment surely brings. Still others are highly dedicated to their professions, and want to devote the time necessary to accomplish their other goals in life. They know that kids are a big commitment of time and energy. People make the decision to live childfree as individuals and as couples, and they happily choose to enjoy their single life or their life as a couple.

Unfortunately, our society makes judgements about the personal choices we make and about our lifestyles. Some people still have a hard time understanding why someone would not want his or her own children. In fact, people can be openly critical about it. Family and friends can make insensitive, judgmental remarks without even stopping to think about their impact on those of us who make this choice. We will address dealing with this more specifically in a later chapter about family and friends and building a support network.

The people who have chosen a life that does not include raising their own children often view their lives as rich, full, exciting, and challenging. They do not believe they need a child to make themselves or their lives complete. This is a viewpoint that is at the opposite end of the spectrum from where we are when we begin infertility treatment. It feels a lifetime away from the beginning of infertility treatment. But it is also a position that ultimately can bring us joy, comfort, and relief depending on what happens to us along the way.

During my interview with Ann I spoke at length with her about her decision to not have children. I asked her to describe some universal themes she finds in the people she works with and concepts she thinks are important for people to know. These thoughts are based on her personal and professional experience as a psychologist. She said: "I think that having kids is a tough road. I don't think that it is such a good idea to adopt if you don't want to take the tough road. I don't think it is really fair to a child if there aren't other strong motivations to adopt. Basically when a child is concerned, you have to make a decision, you have to go this way or that way. You have to think about marching to a different drummer instead of thinking that your life is going to unfold like everybody else's. Those people who choose not to have children have a harder time. I think imagining it is very difficult. You can't imagine. You come from a family so you don't know how life is structured or how it flows involuntarily. I didn't want to adopt and I made a good life."

If you choose to remain childfree, Ann recommends that you "find some other things that you are passionate about that can really give your life a whole lot of meaning. You know that it takes some searching. What is it that is so meaningful to you that it could feel like you did something worthwhile? Parenthood clearly offers that and is a form of that. Can you tolerate being different? Can you tolerate that some people will think that something is wrong with you for not having kids?"

One of the important points that Ann addresses is the idea of finding meaningful things in your life. There are ways you can connect with children, if you decide you still want to be around them in an ongoing way. You may have close friends or family with children and you can play an important role in their lives. Ann spoke with me about the importance of her godparents in her life. She could talk with them about things that she was uneasy speaking with her parents about. We have very close friends who have no children, but who are actively involved in my daughter's life. She loves them and loves spending time with them, and they are very happy to have her be a part of their lives as well. These are strong ties that will remain over the course of their lifetimes and will ultimately enrich all of their lives.

Volunteer work is another effective way to bring new meaning into your life. There are countless organizations such as Big Brothers, Big Sisters, Girl Scouts and Boy Scouts. There are hospitals that welcome volunteers. There are camps and schools or reading and mentoring programs for children available everywhere, and you can find them, if you take the time to look. These are opportunities to have a rich interaction with children and make a difference in their lives. You can do volunteer work that has no connection with children to bring new meaning into your life. You can choose to travel. You can write a book. Some people get more involved in a religious organization, an organization that fights hunger or disease, or one that assists people in other countries. The possibilities are endless. The rewards are very strong as well.

Just as Ann implied, you may need to be creative about the direction that you choose to go. Spend some time thinking about it and see what feels right for you. Give yourself permission to try things, and, if it doesn't work out, go on to something new. Talk to friends and family about people, places, or charitable organizations they may be aware of that could use your help.

Another thing to consider doing is building more personal satisfaction into your own life to make it richer. This may mean spending more time taking care of yourself, or allowing yourself more quality time with the people in your life who are important to you. What I mean by quality time is doing things that you enjoy and that nurture your spirit. You may want to work on improving your own health through exercise. Take time out of your daily routine to pamper yourself in some special way. Make time to do things for yourself that you enjoy. Being childless is a gift of time, and an opportunity to enrich your life in other ways.

One additional thing you can do to help yourself through this process is to talk to others who are going through it or have gone through it. Find out about methods they used to get to this place and how they made this decision. Ask them whether, when they look back, there are any things they might have done in a different way. Find out what worked for them, what gave them strength and support, and helped them get more comfortable with this decision. Ask them if they still have doubts from time to time. How and at what times do their doubts come out? Ask what they do to handle these emotions when they arise. This will also help you to normalize some of the thoughts and feelings you may be having. This is another way to empower yourself through their experience and knowledge.

You can contact your local RESOLVE chapter to see if they have names of other people who have chosen to be childfree that you can contact. RESOLVE can tell you if there are any local groups in your area that have other people who have made a similar choice. You can also contact the Childfree Network. Their address can be found in Chapter 22. There are many other people who have tried infertility treatment and failed and have decided not to pursue surrogacy or adoption.

This is a hard place to be, and it often requires a new beginning. So much is put into pursuing the dream of being parents, and the sacrifices can loom larger when they seem to be in vain. Letting go of these struggles and sacrifices and achieving closure can lead to a new beginning. Often it's helpful to know that others are sharing the difficult transitions of this new life departure. Talking openly with others in the same situation is often healing. Acknowledging the grief that goes with the loss of the dream, and mourning this is an important part of reaching an end. Letting go of the dream, and accepting the pain of that ending, is critical to beginning again and building a rich, new life. This will take time, but your future is open wide with possibility. When the day comes that you are ready to dream again, there will be a whole new fulfilling life you can pursue and make come true.

CHAPTER 11
THE PSYCHOLOGY OF INFERTILITY AND TREATMENT

Because I am a clinical social worker, I take an interest in the psychological issues that arise for people who are dealing with medical problems. I spent many years working with people in hospitals who faced a wide assortment of medical problems and their resulting psychological challenges. Patients commonly have to struggle with psychological issues in order to overcome their medical problems. I am a great believer in the mind and body being linked in ways that are impossible to separate. In the specific area of infertility, there has been a lot of research that shows that fertility can be impacted by stress and depression. For example, research seems to indicate that women who have a history of depression have a higher rate of infertility. Women who were treated for their depression then showed a higher success rate at getting pregnant.

In this chapter I will look at some of the most common emotions that people struggle with when going through infertility problems. My belief is that finding out we have infertility problems makes us feel different from the majority of people, as though our lives can not be "normal." It is helpful to know that the emotional cycles you will go through are shared by many other people. At a time when life is feeling so out of control, it needs to be said that you are not crazy for having these feelings. It is normal to feel intense anger or sadness, as well as the other emotions I will describe. Knowing that this is normal will hopefully empower you. I will give you some useful information that can help you navigate through these waves of feelings, and I will also give you some tools to help you move forward in this journey, whether it leads towards having a child or making the choice to remain childfree.

Many people who undergo infertility treatment have to take medications to regulate their menstrual cycles. These medications also impact hormone levels. Just experiencing infertility on its own merit is enough to cause depression, but the medications needed to fight your infertility can also impact you emotionally. I made reference to some of these medications and their side-effects back in Chapter 3, when I reviewed infertility treatment. You may find that it is difficult to think clearly at times, or you may have mood swings, or you may just not feel like yourself. These can all be side effects of the medications, but another component of this may be depression. You may have headaches or difficulty sleeping as well. All of these factors work together to impact your emotions at this difficult point in your life. Discuss any medications you may be taking with your doctor, and find out if there is the potential for a side effect that can affect you psychologically. If this is the case, talk to your doctor or therapist about how to anticipate, recognize, and cope with these psychological symptoms. You may need to be on these medications for an extended period of time.

By definition a couple is diagnosed as having an infertility problem after unsuccessfully trying to have a child for at least a year. A year is a long time. All of the emotion wrapped up with ongoing and repeated failure, while trying to do something so personal, can be psychologically immobilizing, particularly when you feel you should be able to do it naturally. Having a baby is something so many people all around us do. It appears so easy. Pregnancy is something you plan on, and few of us expect that there will be problems with making this happen. In her article entitled "The Psychological Component of Infertility," Patricia Mahlstedt, Ed.D looks at losses we experience as adults that have the greatest impact on depression and how they relate to infertility treatment. She describes the losses as:

• Loss of a relationship.
• Loss of health.
• Loss of self-esteem.
• Loss of self-confidence.
• Loss of security.
• Loss of a fantasy or the hope of fulfilling an important fantasy.
• Loss of something or someone of great symbolic value.(27)

Dr. Mahlstedt points out in her article any one of these losses by itself is enough to be the precipitant for a situational depression. A situational depression occurs as a result of a trying event that happens in life, which then triggers symptoms of depression such as sadness, loss of sleep, appetite, or inability to enjoy anything. For example, the loss of a job or the death of somebody you know can trigger a situational depression. This is not related to any chemical imbalance. When you think about it, you realize that all of the losses listed by Ms. Mahstedt are associated with the struggle of infertility.

Infertility is a loss that many of us were not expecting. It is hard to prepare yourself for something you don't expect. This initial loss can snowball into many of these other bad feelings. Situational depression can seem all but impossible to avoid, when all of these losses are piled on top of each other. The stresses listed above can become particularly acute when the doctor is not able to identify the reason or reasons for your infertility problem.

While infertility can be stressful on many levels simultaneously, you may find that not all of these feelings of loss apply to you. Or you may feel them at different times, as you move through different aspects of your journey. You should also keep in mind that, if you have a partner, your partner may experience these losses in different ways than you do. Your partner may also cope with them differently. This can create tension and conflict between you. Being aware of this, acknowledging it, and talking about it with your partner may head off potential problems between the two of you. This is another example where educating yourself can become a vehicle for you to take control of your infertility treatment, rather than letting it take control of you and your life.

The media has really latched on to the issue of postpartum depression recently. It is important to recognize that women who have undergone infertility treatment and do have a child may be at more risk for postpartum depression, because all of the attention is now being focused on the new child. Mom was used to having a lot of the attention during her infertility treatment, and, ironically, the mother may now feel some sense of being left out. This combined with the hormonal upheavals of childbirth may result in feelings of depression and sadness.

KEEP YOUR PARTNER ENGAGED

Trying times are when we need our partners to support us. It is common, though, to push our partners away when we are struggling with things. It's important to let them know in advance that you are going to need their help in this process, and that they should be there throughout, whether you ask them to be at the time or not. Get your partner involved at the beginning and ask them to stay engaged—this can be critical to dealing with the roller coaster ride of infertility.

Try to involve your partner as much as possible in the infertility treatment process. Have your partner go to appointments or important marker tests with you. Have your partner meet with and talk with your doctor. Talk with your partner as you go step-by-step through your infertility treatment, and get their input for decisions that you need to make. Your partner may also need to be directly involved in your treatment. For example, your partner may need to give you medication injections. If you decide to share information with family or friends about the infertility treatment, do it together. Have your partner attend educational programs or read material, or speak with other people that are experiencing similar problems. If your partner is a man, it may help him to have another man to talk to and use as a support person and guide to help him get through this process. My husband has helped other men by sharing his experiences with them.

Dr. Mahlstedt goes on to describe the losses articulated above in much greater detail. The loss of relationships can mean many things. It can mean more than the loss of your partner. You may feel the need to separate yourself from friends who are pregnant or have children because it is too painful to be around them. You may want to put distance between yourself and family members who you feel are putting additional pressure on you. You may feel some sense of disappointment or failure in yourself and believe you are letting your family down because of your inability to have a child.

Later in the article, Dr. Mahlstedt goes on to discuss the impact infertility has on sexuality. This is also another type of loss and a change in your relationship with your partner. She writes: "Another aspect of this loss is the loss of sexual spontaneity. Since the course of treatment often requires scheduled sexual intercourse, sex becomes divided into 'sex for love' and 'sex for doctor.' Each month the medical evaluation probes into the couple's sex life and evaluates the frequency of timing of intercourse, thus violating a deep sense of privacy. Constant intrusion into the most intimate aspect's of one's sex life can cause men and women to feel less sexual, avoid sexual activity, and fail to respond sexually in fertile times....As a result of these humiliating encounters, making love becomes a mechanical chore and a painful reminder of the failure to conceive—far removed from earlier loving sexual relationships."(28)

So, among all of the other losses associated with infertility, you can possibly encounter the loss of intimacy, privacy, and potentially the loss of the spontaneous sexual relationship you had with your partner before infertility. You may have to go to the doctor's office immediately after intercourse for tests. The man will likely be asked to give a sperm sample in the doctor's office. He will be sent to a small room with magazines, a TV, and a VCR with pornographic videos. All of these materials are provided in case he needs help producing a sperm sample in this sterile environment. What does all of this do to your self-esteem and your self-confidence? For people who are used to maintaining privacy and control of their personal lives, much of this intrusive process can be a humiliating experience.

COPING WITH LOSS

Dr. Mahlstedt does share ideas about coping with these feelings of loss, and she makes suggestions on how to overcome them. She discusses the strong relationship between grief and loss in her article. She makes a number of recommendations to help people move through this difficult phase of infertility treatment. She makes the following recommendations:

• Couples need to accept differences in feelings and in ways of coping. Although few people see divorce as a consequence of infertility, many couples report increased hostility and anger. This fighting is usually about the other person's feelings or attitude... Couples argue about feelings because they make assumptions about what the other person's feelings mean, do not like assumptions, and so try to change the other's feelings. A couple is two individuals, and to expect both to feel the same about infertility or to express their feeling in the same way causes considerable stress.

- Each person needs to take time to hear how the infertility process is affecting his/her spouse. Listen carefully... If necessary, couples can set aside a specific amount of time each day (10-30 minutes) to talk about feelings. Some may set a timer and stop when the time is over. Of course, this routine is not to be used on a day when the couple gets especially discouraging news.

- Each person needs to take responsibility for his/her feelings, knowing that only he can determine what kind of support he needs and when and from whom he needs it. Likewise, feeling responsible for taking away a spouse's pain is fruitless. One can only listen and be supportive. The other person must make the changes.

- Couples must nurture their marriage. They can learn to live for what is present and not for what is missing in their relationship. They can go out on dates and talk about the love they feel for each other. Having fun and creating a balance between the sadness of infertility and the joy of being married lessens the burden.

- Some couples might want to take a vacation from the day-to-day struggles of infertility. A 'time-out' can make it easier to see infertility as just a part of their lives and can enable them to see times ahead when work for pregnancy will be over...

- Couples must share with others and ask for what they need from them. They must widen support systems and broaden their bases of information.

- Very importantly, each couple must be reasonable in their expectations. No one can take away the realities of life that cause pain.(29)

Dr. Mahlstedt has a lot of experience and knowledge in working with people who have undergone infertility treatment. She also trains other healthcare professionals who work with people who undergo infertility treatment. This particular article was written for healthcare professionals, but I thought her comments were very useful for people who were not necessarily medical or healthcare professionals. Her last recommendation really relates to the issue of having to deal with the day-to-day realities that we have to face in our lives. We will see pregnant women on the street and in television and magazine ads showing happy families. I am sure you have your own personal list of things that you see and hear on a regular basis that can be a source of pain for you, as you continue on your path through infertility treatment.

One common thread that all these recommendations share is the notion that ongoing infertility is linked with grief. Many people have a theory that the feelings we experience as a result of infertility are very similar to the stages of feelings people go through as they try to deal with death and dying. The difference with infertility of course is that we may never have a child to mourn. People still need to go through the rituals necessary to mourn this very significant loss. This is the only way we can begin to move ahead with our lives and determine what the next step may be for us. It is helpful to take a look at the stages of death and dying and make these valuable comparisons.

Dr. Elizabeth Kubler-Ross is famous for her work with people who were dying and her insights helped their families. Her belief was that, as people were coping with death and dying, they went through stages of grief. She also believed it was an ongoing process. The Five Stages are: Denial, Anger, Bargaining, Depression, and Acceptance. You can probably see the parallels when comparing these stages to the stages we go through when struggling with infertility issues. I think it is useful to look at these stages more carefully. The first thing to understand about these stages is that you may find yourself returning to one more than once, and they may not necessarily occur in this order. You may be in one stage a long time and another may have a short duration. Just view this scenario of progression as a guide, and use the elements that may apply to you.

THE INITIAL STAGES OF GRIEF

The first stage is one of denial and isolation. We usually don't anticipate we will be infertile unless there is a family history, a known medical problem, or we start trying to have a child much later in life. Otherwise, there is an assumption that, when you want to have a child and start trying, it will happen. Often, it is only after a long period of trying to conceive a child that disbelief turns into denial, shock, or surprise. Frequently, people will intentionally put off having a child, while they pursue career choices or wait to find the right partner. They may also wait for financial reasons or other reasons. In these cases, they are making a conscious choice to not have a child and then a conscious decision to have a child. There is an inherent assumption that things will go according to plan. With the more extensive media coverage around infertility, we are beginning to realize that is not always the case.

Barbara Eck Manning describes denial in these terms: "Denial is a protective defense mechanism which is appropriate to sudden and overwhelming events. It is not successful as a long term defense mechanism, and it should break down in the face of reality to give way to the normal and necessary feelings to come."(30) In the denial stage you will continue to try all avenues possible to have a child and truly believe that, if you continue, something will work. You don't want to leave any stone unturned. If one doctor tells you that you really don't have much of a chance of successfully conceiving a child, you may choose to go to another doctor, until you hear what you want to hear.

Ms. Manning points out that denial can be a healthy defense mechanism to initially get you through a traumatic event, but eventually you must move beyond it at some point. If you don't, the denial will begin to cause dysfunction in other areas of your life. It may negatively impact close relationships because you feel other people don't understand you or they don't share your feelings. Denial may lead you to try to mask your painful feelings, but they will manifest themselves in other ways. For example, anger may become internalized and turn into depression. As Ms. Manning suggests, at some point you need to open yourself up to these strong feelings in order to begin to move forward on another path that you can choose.

I already have made reference to isolation. As you struggle with infertility issues, when you learn that having a child may not happen, you may feel that you don't want to be around other people, especially those who have children. This is a very normal response. Sue and Howard, the egg donor couple, spoke to me about this. Howard told me: "Sue didn't want to go to my friends' birthday parties. So I really couldn't go either. They all knew what was going on. Most of them understood. What's funny is we have a lot of friends who were trying to have kids at the same time as us. Then they would have kids. It would definitely impact us. Then our relationship with them would drift. That would happen many times."

Sue told me about one friend. "I couldn't go to her son's birthday party," she said. "She was so understanding and wonderful about it and that was really great. I still feel really bad about it, that I couldn't be there for her. These were really important occasions but I just couldn't do it." Sue told me she did talk with her friend as it was happening, and she was fine with it. It is important, when appropriate, to let family and friends know why you may appear to be withdrawing and isolating yourself. I will be talking more about ways to deal with family and friends in the next chapter.

One way to break the isolation pattern is to stay in touch with people you do feel comfortable with—or ask them to stay in touch with you, if you do withdraw. Often, just sharing the story of your burden with others can help relieve the weight of it. You may also have friends that are having their own personal crisis at the same time you are. Sometimes helping a friend deal with their problems will give you the opportunity to not focus on your own problems, and helping others can often offer you some temporary relief. You may have some helpful advice for your friend, and by engaging and giving it, you end up feeling better about yourself, because you are able to help out somebody else. It can be a positive experience for all concerned.

You may find it is hard to go to work and be around people, especially when they are talking about their kids or celebrating a colleague's new baby. That happened to me, while I was working. I couldn't talk to anybody at work about it. But when I went home, I did talk with a friend about it, so I could let some of those feelings out. I was at work when I got the telephone call and found out that my first attempt at trying to get pregnant had failed. All I wanted to do was to leave and go home and crawl under the covers in my bed. But what I did was take a short break and go outside, cry a bit, take some slow, deep breaths, and then I went back to my desk and did my job. If your situation at work is one where people there are aware you are dealing with infertility issues, then be honest with them. If you can, talk with your supervisor or boss about your needs in these situations, and don't be afraid to take time off when you need to.

Guilt is an area I have discussed in previous chapters. It is something many of us experience. Ann, who chose to not have a child, explored the guilt she felt because her parents lost most of their family when they escaped the Holocaust. Ann wanted to bring more people into her family and continue the family line, and assumed that a decision not to have kids would be difficult for her parents to accept. Later, when she spoke with her parents about it, she was very happy to learn that they did not have any of the feelings she feared they would. Ann put off this conversation, but in the end she was glad when she finally talked with her parents directly.

Guilt makes some people feel that they have caused their own infertility. They feel that, because they did something they perceive as bad or wrong in the past, their current state of infertility is the payback for this. We all want to come up with a specific reason to explain to ourselves and others why we find ourselves in a situation that we don't want to be in. This type of irrational thinking, however, just perpetuates your sense of guilt and blame and will prohibit you from moving forward.

Barbara Eck Manning explains, "First people do not control all aspects of life, however much they would like to; second life is not always fair, finally, worthiness and fertility are not related. I finally got to the point where I realized that pregnancy is not a reward for worthiness. Worthiness is its own reward."(31)

These types of feelings can also directly impact your own fertility. I described earlier the research about stress impacting fertility and this is another example of how that can happen. In situations where one person is identified as the reason for the infertility, there may be feelings of guilt, or one partner in moments of anger or frustration may blame the other for their inability to help conceive a child.

What Ann did is really the key to getting through this stage, that is: talk to the people close to you or the person or persons you may be lashing out at. You may find that some of the feelings of guilt that you have are self-inflicted and the other person does not have the feelings you think they do.

The other critical way you can help yourself to get through this stage is to attend a support group where other people are going through infertility. I am certain you will hear about guilt as a universal theme, and that others will talk about it. Find out all the ways other people in the group got through it. Just hearing them share their stories will help you to realize you are not alone and that these feelings you have are not uncommon. Some people don't feel comfortable in a group setting. If the guilt and blame stage does linger on to the point that it is significantly impacting your relationships with other people or other areas of your life, then you should consider seeing an individual counselor. A good counselor can help guide you through this difficult time and offer you some good ideas about coping mechanisms you can use to heal yourself.

OTHER STAGES OF GRIEF

Loss of control is one of the most difficult feelings to go through. It has components of anger, rage, depression, and feelings of hopelessness. The anger you feel may be at yourself, at your body for failing you, and at other people. Some of these people may have done nothing but have children, when you can't. You may have anger towards your doctor and other healthcare professionals you have been working with. There may be anger directed towards your partner, if that person has been diagnosed with the infertility problem, or if they don't seem supportive enough. You may experience anger if a medical problem is not diagnosed, and you never know why you can't conceive a child. You may also feel anger and rage at your family or friends for comments they make, or things they do or don't do that may feel insensitive. You also could be angry at yourself for waiting too long to begin having a child. The list can go on and on. Think about what fits for you.

Bargaining is something many of us do when we find ourselves in a situation that feels painful and unbearable. It is a natural human response. For example, if we find ourselves in a position where we are unable to have a child, and we have repeated failed attempts, we may fall back on our faith. We might promise God, or whatever higher power we may believe in, that if we are fortunate enough to have a child, we will be the best possible parent we can be. I remember promising myself that if I was lucky enough to have a child I would do volunteer work for RESOLVE, since they had helped me through my infertility process. You may make agreements with your partner, saying: "If we just try this one more time, I won't ask for anything else again." I am sure you can come up with your own examples. The point is we try to bargain, to make an agreement, sometimes silently to ourselves, and we promise to do whatever it takes to get to the ultimate goal of pregnancy and a healthy baby. If we do achieve this goal, sometimes it can be difficult to keep these promises we made. However, when you are attempting to have a child, you truly feel in your heart that you will do anything you have to do to have a successful pregnancy and a healthy child.

Anger that is internalized becomes depression. I think it is fair to say that most of us who experience some type of infertility problem also have to deal with some form of anger and depression. For some of us, the intensity and frequency of the depression may be greater, and for some the depression can become more disabling and immobilize us in other areas of our lives. Feeling angry, depressed or sad about not being able to have a child is a natural reaction. Symptoms of depression include crying, loss of appetite, ongoing fatigue, loss of interest in things you ordinarily care about, and an inability to get any joy or happiness out of anything. If you are struggling, you do need to monitor your symptoms, and keep a close eye on how your feelings are impacting your day to day activities, your relationships, and your ability to function.

If your ability to function on a day-to-day basis does seem to be impaired, and if this goes on for any extended period of time, you definitely should consider seeing a mental health professional or perhaps a psychiatrist. Dr. Richard Marrs, author of *The Fertility Book*, offers some pointers on how to stop this wave of depression when it becomes debilitating. He says it is critical not to run from these feelings, but to face them directly. He says the best way to achieve this is to do the following:

- Acknowledge and accept your feelings. Don't judge them. They are the way you feel.
- Allow yourself to really feel what is hurting you. Don't black it out.
- Talk about your feeling with someone. Your spouse, a close family member or friend, a therapist, or a support group
- Discuss the use of antidepressant medications with your doctor. Short term use may be of help to you.(32)

I want to comment on his last point about medications. If antidepressant medication is indicated, it should be monitored and administered by a psychiatrist. It is also really important that you let your fertility doctor know that you are on an antidepressant. Let your fertility doctor know the medication and the dose, and any doctor you see should be aware of all medications you are taking, including those related to infertility treatment. Sometimes one medication can interact with another medication causing a negative side effect. You should consult with your doctors if you are experiencing severe depression. You and your doctors will need to determine the severity of the depression. Your doctor may recommend that you take a break from your fertility treatment while the depression is being treated. In fact, sometimes taking a break from the fertility treatment is the best thing you can do. A break can help you get more grounded and focused on things other than infertility. It can give a chance to step back and determine what the best next-step is for you. And, as I stated earlier, relieving depression may be necessary to the success of any additional fertility treatment you undergo.

The final stage of grieving is acceptance. Acceptance does not mean that you are happy with the way things are. Acceptance does mean that you figure out ways to continue your life in a meaningful way. It does not mean that you are ignoring the loss, forgetting about the loss, or not grieving the loss. When I worked with rehabilitation patients, people who suffered life changing medical problems such as stroke, brain injuries, or amputations, we would often speak about stages of loss. I felt more comfortable using the word adaptation rather than acceptance.

When you deal with infertility, your life has changed in a dramatic way, and it will impact the way you view yourself and your world forever. But that is not to say that you cannot find ways to do the things that are important to you. You may need to bring new things and new people into your life to help give it meaning. The struggle may lead you to approach the things you do in a different way with a fresh perspective. The intensity of the pain that you feel will begin to diminish with time. There will be ups and downs, but if you use some of the guidelines outlined throughout this book, they can help you get through this difficult period. You know yourself better than anybody else, and you will know what works for you and what does not.

One thing that may be helpful as you go through this process is keeping a journal. Sometimes, writing a letter to say goodbye to your unborn child or the life you might have had as a biological parent can help, too. You might like to try using some other type of art, if that is a way you feel more comfortable expressing your feelings. These are all ways of letting your emotions out. It is important to have an outlet as you go through these stages of grieving. Sometime we don't have anybody in our lives we feel we can discuss our innermost thoughts and feelings with. You may be afraid of releasing these emotions in front of another person. You may not feel comfortable putting people in a position where they are expected to be there for you, especially if they are not capable of supporting you in this way. These other outlets for self-expression are safe, and they can be a good reference point for you, as you work through the process of coping with infertility.

KNOWING AND HEALING OURSELVES

Maintaining a strong, positive sense of our identity is the thing we all want to work towards, in spite of what may happen to us in our infertility journey. Lara Devereaux and Ann Jackoway Hammerman address this critical issue in their book, *Infertility and Identity: New Strategies for Treatment.* In this book they look at ways we can get a healthy identity back as we battle infertility. They outline "four key elements" people use in the process of integrating infertility and identity. These elements include:

- Recognizing that infertility is a condition and not a definition of self.
- Experiencing grief and accepting that healing comes from allowing themselves to experience the full range of their emotions.
- Knowing that they can proactively manage their response to infertility.
- Acknowledging that infertility will forever change their feelings about marriage and parenthood and their negotiation of the remaining stages of life.(33)

I believe their elements are very insightful. We get so wrapped up in our infertility treatment that it becomes all-encompassing, and we can't separate it from any other aspects of ourselves. Infertility is one aspect of who you are, but we are made up of many parts. Allowing ourselves to be vulnerable to the many emotions that emerge through the infertility journey can be a terrifying prospect. It can also ultimately be a rich experience, in the sense that you can learn new things about yourself, your partner, and perhaps your family and friends. You can gain a greater understanding of yourself. Perhaps, you will surprise yourself in terms of what you are able to endure. You may emerge a stronger person.

The final element of acknowledging that infertility changes us forever is also very important. Whether we are ultimately successful in having a child or not, we will be forever changed. People who are parents after infertility do have some differences from people who never struggled with this. I will address this in "Parenting after Infertility" in Chapter 14. People who ultimately do not have a child through infertility treatment are also clearly changed forever. If you have this experience, it will affect the choices you make about the next stage of your life, and how you feel about these choices in the future. Though this loss is painful, with acceptance, it can also become a source of growth and renewal.

Just as the physical and medical pieces of infertility treatment assume a roller coaster pattern, our emotions and feelings will also be on a parallel path, with many ups and downs. The guidelines and models that are addressed in this chapter will hopefully give you the tools you need to help get a better handle on this roller coaster. There are ways to take control of the psychological components of infertility. Ultimately, you will certainly emerge a different person, but hopefully stronger, too. One of the keys to coping more effectively with the infertility journey is to develop a strong support network. How do we deal with our family and friends? Where can we go when we need additional support while struggling with infertility? How do we ask for help? These are some of the questions that will be addressed in the next chapter.

CHAPTER 12
BUILDING A SUPPORT NETWORK

I grew up in a household where family was extremely important. We build our relationships with our families from the day we are born. Behaviors and personalities are shaped within the family system, and they can stay with us throughout our lives. That can be a good thing or a bad thing, depending on what kind of a relationship you have with your parents, siblings, aunts and uncles, and extended family. We often allow our families to do and say things to us that we would never permit anybody else to do or say. It's because they are our family. The bonds are strong. The imprint of your family relationships is there, whether your family is a part of your life or not. We often assume a role early on in our family system, and that role stays with us throughout our lifetimes, unless we make a conscious choice to change it.

Now you find yourself undergoing infertility treatment. You want and need support to help you get through this experience. There may be things you are unable to say to your partner for fear of upsetting him or her. There are feelings and thoughts you need to share, but where do you turn? In the last chapter, we looked at the feelings of isolation that stem from struggling with infertility, and acknowledged you need to do what you can to avoid having this happen to you. You may be dealing with periods of moodiness, anger, sadness, or frustration as you go through the infertility process. Your family or friends may provide a safe haven to let some of these feelings out.

On the other hand, your family or friends may not feel like a safe place to talk about these issues. What if you have a sibling, friend, or in-law who is pregnant? You may have a sibling or in-law who has several children, and who seemed to get pregnant easily, as planned. How will talking with them or being around them make you feel? There can be some difficulty and discomfort associated with being around a family member or friend who is pregnant, or who has children, when you are dealing with infertility treatment. You may not be emotionally available to celebrate these moments of parenting with them.

The first thing you need to think about is: how much information do you want to share with your family and friends about your infertility treatment? Who do you want to tell? Who do you want them to tell? Spend some thinking about how specific you want to get about what you are doing. Consider how many details you want to share about each step of your treatment. How frequently do you want to talk to your family and friends about where things are at with your treatment? At what stage of your treatment do you want to give them this information? Who will be sharing the information, you or your partner?

In answering these questions, it is helpful to imagine some of the effects this information may have on people. For example, imagine how knowing about your infertility treatment might impact your family's relationships with your unborn child. In a similar context, consider what impact knowing about your infertility treatment will have on their relationship with you. There can be religious issues to consider as well. Some people have strong opinions about infertility treatment, based on their religious or ethical belief systems. These are all very personal decisions. There is no right or wrong answer. But you will need to be sensitive to the opinion of others in deciding how open to be, and in considering this, remember you are looking for support.

You do need to discuss how open to be with your partner, so that you both come to the same decision about it. When my husband and I spoke about this, his bias was to be totally open and tell everybody about it. My opinion was that most people did not need to know the specifics about what we were doing and how it was going. Often, the appropriate disclosure choice is the one that both partners can agree to follow, and there should be a mutually understood expectation around disclosure. My husband and I ultimately decided to tell our immediate family and some very close friends.

Disclosure to family and friends is one of the toughest issues associated with infertility treatment. In addition to our own feelings about this, there is another critical piece of disclosure that you need to think carefully about, and this is the fact that what you tell others will eventually get back to your child. We struggled with this a lot and continue to struggle with it. So does everybody else who has undergone infertility treatment. RESOLVE does seminars around disclosure issues. These seminars are extremely helpful. I strongly recommend them. I will address the disclosure issue in much greater detail in Chapter 17. This is such an important and complicated issue that it merits a chapter of its own.

COMMUNICATING WITH PEOPLE

When considering who to tell and what to say, remember how you felt when you first began delving into the infertility world. Everything was new, somewhat unknown, perhaps scary. Use this as a guide, when you think about how it will all feel for your family and friends, if you tell them. Some may have had experience with this. Others may not. I was surprised to learn how many people have had the experience of a miscarriage or some other type of problem with pregnancy. When I had my miscarriage, I was really surprised at the number of people who came to my husband and me to share their experiences as a means of offering us support.

We can all relate to stories about insensitive comments people make about getting pregnant—statements like, "Just relax, it will happen," or, "Maybe you are just trying too hard," or,"Why don't you have any kids yet, you aren't getting any younger?" The list goes on and on. Eliza told me about a striking example of a friend she had who was not at all aware of the impact of her comments. Eliza said: "Some of our friends were awful. I mean totally insensitive. One friend's father was a well-known doctor and I felt I couldn't turn to my friend for any-thing, because I would get her father's advice on top of it. There was an infamous dinner, where they sat around and talked about another friend of ours who was having problems, and I basically walked out of the restaurant and vowed never to have dinner with these friends again. Of course, I changed my mind shortly afterwards. About four months later, I let my friend have it. She said something and I went off and told her she was the most insensitive person on Earth."

Todd quickly added: "There were people who just didn't realize what a sensitive topic it was, and the fact that we were trying and it didn't happen for a long time was really personally difficult. I think if you are not going through it, it's difficult to understand how emotionally frustrating it can be." Todd went on to describe his family's reaction. He told me: "My family was actually very supportive. It was only towards the end, as we realized we had to get a little more aggressive, that their biases and opinions started to come through a little more—to the effect that: 'You are throwing good money after bad, and why don't you give up and adopt a kid already?'"

Sue and Howard also shared their experiences with friends and family. Howard told me: "Well, the choice was: we started telling people about what we were doing, and they asked the same questions over and over, [so] we stopped, basically. It was kind of weird. Here we give speeches on it and I never told my closest friends. I think I went as far as saying IVF. People would think it was strange." Not everyone has the expectation that you should talk to them about infertility. Some people consider this a highly private part of life, and these people can include your family and friends.

Sue added, "I think the whole family and friends thing was like an arc. Like [fertility treatment] started out: you are just trying these minimally invasive things, but you don't talk about that. You just talk about: 'We are trying to get pregnant and start a family.' Then you talk, [and] it is more like a bell curve. It begins to get more stressful, and then I wanted to get it off my chest. But then it got to the point that, every time I would talk to somebody, I felt like I would have to educate them and inform them about all of these acronyms and medical treatments. I remember all of the emotional, moral, ethical, legal, and financial implications of all of this stuff. It got to the point where I could not tell everybody all of this stuff anymore. So then I started going down the other side, until I got more closed, and at the end I only spoke to a support group about it. It was exhausting talking to people about that."

Deciding how much to tell people depends on their ability to absorb the information and how much time is reasonable to spend "educating" them in the process. Not everyone wants to take the time to learn about all the issues. Other people want to explore every detail, and as Sue said, this too, can be exhausting. Striking a balance can be hard to do, and the process reveals a lot about our relationships with others. Sue added: "I learned a lot about my friends and who really tried to understand, and who was scared and didn't want to hear about that stuff, and who was afraid it might impact them personally—and just people who were so self-absorbed that they didn't have the time to care about that stuff. I really weeded some people out of my life at that time."

If you talk with different couples, you will hear stories about friends and family who were incredibly caring, and others who were seemingly insensitive. Some people, as Todd said, will even try to impose their values and biases on you. There are steps you can take to gain some control over some of these outcomes. The key is for you to educate people about what your needs are. It may seem tough to take the energy to do this at a time when you feel you have no extra energy to spare. However, in the long run this can be of enormous help to you and the other important people in your life. Let them know what's happening, but most of all tell them what they can do to support you.

Often, the important people in your life are as uncomfortable as you are in the initial stages of communication. They know you are going through a difficult time, but they don't know what to say or do. They don't know what you need. The amount of support and help you will get back depends on you laying the groundwork for this. You need to think about what you need and how people can help you. Building a support network can be very gratifying for all concerned. You can end up strengthening bonds that were there and learning new things about the importance of the people that are close to you. If your family and friends choose to ignore the requests you make, then you always have the option of putting some distance between you and them, at least during this emotionally-charged time.

HELPING OTHERS UNDERSTAND

In both of the cases discussed above, the couples did not let their family and friends know what they needed. They were emotionally drained and reacted to what was said or not said by their family and friends. Hopefully by laying this foundation early on, you will avoid some of these painful episodes and gain strength from the people around you. Relationships can be a source of comfort and support with good communication. But even the best relationships can seem to take away what little energy you have if you don't open up and ask for help and understanding. The important people in our lives want to be there for us, and we have to let them know how to do this.

In the back of her pamphlet, "Understanding: A guide to Impaired Fertility for Family and Friends," Ms. Johnston has written some very helpful information that you can use as a roadmap to share with your family and friends. Her list of twelve points includes the following:

- Do be ready to listen when one or the other partner or both need to talk. Don't, however, offer unsolicited advice unless you are absolutely sure both that your advice is factual and needed and that you are prepared for the possibility of being seen as a meddler.
- Do be sensitive. Infertility is a very personal issue and is very important to most couples whom it affects. Don't joke about it or minimize it in any way.
- Do let the couple know that you realize that infertility can be a difficult problem and that you care about them.
- Do be patient. The infertile couple's two week cycles of hope followed by disappointment may bring mood swings.
- Do be flexible. At some point couples will find child-centered activities welcome and will want to be involved. At other times they may need to be allowed to isolate themselves. Don't impose your own behavioral expectations on them.
- Do be realistic. Don't continue to deny the problem or its diagnosis in an attempt to be kind or optimistic. Support the decision to take time out from treatment or to stop it entirely.
- Do be supportive. Having satisfied yourself that the couple has access to expert medical care as it is defined by a support and advocacy organization, don't impugn their decision-making abilities by implying that you know a better doctor. Don't put down the couple's chosen treatment or alternative.

- Do be truthful. Don't try to hide your own pregnancy or that of another friend or family member out of 'kindness.' Instead respect the infertile couple's need to be told as others are learning of it and try to acknowledge, privately, that you know that the pregnancy may be difficult for them at times and you are willing to be understanding of this.
- Do be an advocate. As you hear other family members and friends react to the infertile couple insensitively, educate those other 'carers' to the pain of infertility.
- Do let the couple know if you are finding it difficult to know what to say rather than saying nothing at all when you can't find the right words.
- Do remember that infertility is a highly individual condition. When, how, and if the infertile couple reacts to its issues and stages will depend largely on their own circumstances. It is not at all abnormal for some reactions to be severe. These people are grieving.
- Do recommend RESOLVE, IAAC, and groups like them to the couple who may not be aware of them. Consider as well that such volunteer-run and donation-supported organizations need your financial support as well as the memberships of infertile couples and the professionals that work with them if they are to continue to be able to provide a full range of services.(34)

I think Ms. Johnston has done a wonderful job of laying out a roadmap for you to seek support. You can use this list of suggestions as a tool with your family and friends. You can share it with them, or review it and share the aspects that are important to you. Consider this list carefully and outline what things family and friends can do to help you through your infertility journey. You may have additional things that you want to add or aspects of this list you want to emphasize as potential pitfall areas. Different parts may apply to different people, so think about how these ideas relate to the individuals in your life. You may want to ask different people to do different things, or you may need to define specific boundaries for some people but not for others.

If you do not feel comfortable saying these things to your

family and friends, then recruit a trusted friend or your partner to share this information with them. You may even want to have it written down. In the event that communication breaks down at some point, you can use this list as a reference for them and refer to it as a means of reminding them of what you need. Remember, information you share with people should be consistent. The story should stay the same, though you can tell it to varying degrees of detail, depending on what's appropriate with a given individual. You should be clear about this with any intermediary. Trust depends on honesty, and inconsistencies in the story you tell people will eventually surface and can impact your relationships. This doesn't mean that you have to express the same needs to everyone. In fact, it is appropriate that you need different things from different people. Letting individual people know what in particular you need from them is the key to building an effective support network.

GETTING SUPPORT

When you review the bullet points above you can see it is an extensive list that asks for ongoing sensitivity, understanding, and support from your family and friends. Successful relationships take a lot of effort from everybody involved. There are some things you need to be willing to do in order to help build a lasting, successful, support network. This may be hard for you given the emotional and physical demands that your infertility treatment will make on you. But the rewards will be great.

Be honest and open with family and friends about what is going on with you physically and emotionally when you feel it is appropriate. You cannot expect them to read your mind. Give your family and friends information that will help them gain insight about your treatment and how it will affect you physically and emotionally. Try to be flexible with the people closest to you, since you will be demanding flexibility from them. If you have a blow up or an unpleasant exchange, give yourself some time to gain perspective about what and why it happened. Try to go back and address it. Don't leave things hanging and words unspoken. Try to pull back a bit, if possible, to think about how your situation is affecting family and friends. They will appreciate that you are making the effort to do this. It can make a huge difference. It will also alleviate some of your stress, knowing that they are aware of what you need. Sometimes, nothing works better than having a pathway for discussion outlined in advance, so that, in the event of a communication breakdown, you know how to move forward. Few things are as stressful as unresolved conflict.

I want to spend some time talking about holidays, which can be a major problem for people who are undergoing infertility treatment. Your family members, and perhaps your special friends, will often have implicit expectations that you will automatically be attending holiday celebrations such as Christmas, Thanksgiving, birthdays, weddings, anniversaries, etc. Mothers Day and Fathers Day can be incredibly painful times for people who have lost children or who have been unsuccessful at having a child. There are commercials on TV and in magazines. Cards and displays are all over shopping malls and in the grocery stores. People at workplaces usually celebrate holidays in some way as well. How do you deal with all this? There are some things you can do to manage your way through this issue.

Sometimes you just have to say no to these invitations. If you know that it will be too painful to participate in a family gathering where lots of kids will be (or a pregnant relative), just tell the person throwing the gathering that you will not be able to attend. If you have implemented the roadmap previously discussed, they should be accepting and empathetic about your feelings. You might want to arrange another time where you can visit with some of the family or friends you missed seeing at this particular function. You can also make other plans that might just include you and your partner or a couple of other close family or friends.

The holidays often feel burdensome, but they don't have to be that way. We need special times in our lives, especially when we are struggling with a particular issue like infertility. Plan a celebration that will be special for you. You may want to take a memorable vacation at that time of year, going somewhere unusual where you and your partner can have some time alone. Create new traditions that offer you some relief and comfort. Make a really great meal. See a play or a movie. Find new ways to re-energize yourself. Treat yourself or reconnect with others on an intimate level. If big gatherings seem too difficult to deal with, you shouldn't hesitate to decline when you feel that way. If a big work party is going on, for example, you can always tell them you have another function you must attend. You can also choose to attend larger gatherings with the idea that, if it gets too difficult, you can leave early. You may want to discuss this ahead of time with your family or friends, so they are prepared if you decide to make an early exit. Allow yourself some time alone and time to just relax. This will help alleviate the stresses associated with the holidays.

Some people choose to do volunteer work on holidays as a way of coping with their personal losses. It helps take their mind off some of the day-to-day pressures they are struggling with. Volunteering to help other people can re-energize you. I know of people who choose to buy Christmas presents for underprivileged kids. They have decided that, since they can't do this for their own children, they would like to give to other kids. Many people give of themselves during the holidays and assist children who don't have as many opportunities available to them. Gift giving is a common way to participate in the generosity of spirit in this special season. This can be a particularly powerful way for people struggling with infertility to celebrate a holiday like Christmas, Hanukah, or Kwanza.

Gift giving is a symbolic act, and your gift can be large or small. It can be given anonymously or directly, depending on what feels right to you. Giving is an act of compassion that we can be particularly called to during the holidays. Sometimes we can feel obligated by what we've done in the past to mark the holiday. Giving the larger gift of your time through volunteer work is good, if it doesn't add stress to your life. Know what is right for you to do now and only give what you can. Don't feel obligated—the same is true for traditional family or religious celebrations. Missing a year does not put an end to these things, and you will be able to do them again in the future. Giving what you can now is a very fruitful process, and knowing that you will be able to give more again in the future can help you accept your current limits.

In addition to the holidays, another challenging area is setting boundaries. Family, friends, and even associates often make invalid assumptions about what your boundaries are, and then ask you inappropriate questions. You and your partner need to spend some time thinking about how you will handle this when it occurs. People who are not aware of your roadmap of rules, or who choose not to honor it, will step over the line. You may feel your privacy is being invaded or the nature of their questions just doesn't feel right to you. Trust your gut and think it through. You always have the option of saying: "I don't really feel comfortable answering that question." Fill in the blanks. Whatever feels right to you is the message you should try to share with these people. Do give it some thought ahead of time so you won't be caught off guard if this should occur.

Dr. Linda Mintle, in her article "When Families Let You Down", in the RESOLVE of Virginia newsletter of April, 1996, has some good thoughts on how to measure the support you get from your family. She breaks it down into three areas:

- Cohesiveness—the degree of commitment, help provided from one member to the next.
- Expressiveness—the extent to which family members speak out and make their own decisions.
- Conflict—the openness of expressed anger and conflict in a family. Families high on cohesion and expression and lower on conflict are considered supportive.(35)

You know your family well and you may be able to anticipate some of their responses as you ask them to support you through your infertility journey. I include friends in this category, too, since some friendships are like family ties. This is a new realm for you and it will be for them, too. Don't necessarily make assumptions based on past incidents and behaviors. Giving family and friends good information coupled with the guidelines we reviewed above can ultimately lead to stronger connections than you might ever have imagined. Many people I know, and others I have spoken with, were very pleasantly surprised by how helpful and supportive their friends and family members turned out to be. Seeking, generating, and enabling that support network can be one of the most positive experiences to come out of infertility treatment.

CHAPTER 13
PREGNANT AT LAST

Many of us have spent every waking moment during our struggle against infertility thinking and imagining only one thing: a successful pregnancy and a healthy baby. We have all dreamt of the day we would learn that we are pregnant and imagined that feeling of utter joy and ecstasy when we hear the good news. We assume that feeling will continue for the next nine months. Instead, those of us who have battled infertility may find ourselves with a mixture of feelings, including happiness, guilt, awe, hope, anxiety, fear, joy, and possibly even sadness. Nobody prepares us for this. I know it caught me off guard.

There are things that separate those of us who are fortunate enough to get pregnant after infertility from those that get pregnant the old-fashioned way. After I had my baby, I was the leader for a group called PAL (Pregnant at Last). These groups are for the men and women who are lucky enough to get pregnant through infertility treatment. Many of us have ongoing anxiety, health issues, and concerns that something will still go wrong. Many of us fear we will not end up with a healthy child. I only wish a group like this had been available when I got pregnant.

There are a number of universal themes that came up as I led this group. First, couples feel incredible anxiety about their pregnancy. Many of them have experienced failed pregnancies in the past. Their fears can be particularly intense in the first trimester, and for many these fears remain throughout the pregnancy. People who have experienced the ups and downs of infertility treatment will sometimes steel themselves by anticipating that something can and will go wrong. This anticipatory fear prepares them to take on the potential future pain of failure, but it also causes them to live with unnecessary anxiety.

You can find this anxiety in many little things. For example, I can remember how I stalled about getting maternity clothes. I had started showing and the things I could wear from my regular wardrobe were getting more and more limited, yet I wouldn't go shopping. Why was I stalling? When I examined my feelings, I realized that I was terrified to buy maternity clothes because I was fearful of having a miscarriage. If that happened, I felt it would be more painful to face having those clothes and losing my baby. When my mother-in-law called and offered to take me shopping for maternity clothes, I was incredibly fearful. Buying the clothes meant that I believed everything was going to be all right, and I wasn't emotionally prepared to make that leap of faith. I wasn't able to share those feelings with anybody at the time. I also thought that I was the only one that felt this way, but I was wrong.

What can we do about these feelings? There are several options you have. First, it is important to recognize and understand that these feelings are completely normal, and almost everybody who goes through infertility treatment has them in one way or another. Second, you can recognize that you have a choice. You can continue to feel hopeless and ask yourself, *How am I going to get through the next nine months?* Or you can choose to break your pregnancy down into milestones and segments. For example, you can say to yourself, *The baby and I are healthy after eight weeks.* Acknowledging and celebrating milestones can help defuse and counterbalance the fears. Think of milestones such as your first ultrasound, finishing your first trimester, or feeling your baby move for the first time. Pick and choose those events that are meaningful to you and enjoy and celebrate them. I can't tell you how many women I have talked to who have told me they never allowed themselves to celebrate or enjoy their pregnancies because of these fears. Without exception, once their babies were born, they looked back with regret on this.

Once we learn we are pregnant we are caught in between the "fertile world" and the "infertile world." We feel a sense of guilt about counting on the same friends and support networks we relied on while we were going through infertility treatment. Often, when we are in treatment, we share the ups and downs with others in the same boat. After we get pregnant, some of the people in our support network may still be trying to get pregnant, and we have a heightened sensitivity to the mixture of feelings they may have about our successful treatment. We know how hard it is, waiting and hoping to achieve this goal. With other family and friends who have supported us, we can feel guilty because we made a crisis out our infertility, and now our treatment has been successful. They probably assured us it would be successful all along. And now we still have ongoing feelings of anxiety and worry that others may perceive this as unreasonable, too. After we get pregnant, a sense of guilt can cause us to pull away from our support networks. This is another difficult transition that nobody prepares us for.

One of the women in my PAL group told me a story that emphasized this point. She had been going to an infertility clinic affiliated with a hospital. Once she got pregnant, she was referred to an obstetrician at that hospital. The hospital had placed the infertility patients right next to the patients that were coming in for their obstetrical check ups. She felt a tremendous amount of guilt and sadness every time she passed that waiting area with all those infertility patients. We couldn't believe the insensitivity of that hospital, and that they didn't recognize that this system was a problem for many of their patients.

In addition to our own reactions, sometimes the people around us don't understand why we are still struggling with our infertility anxieties. People who have not had infertility problems do not understand the concerns and fears that we commonly experience in relation to our pregnancies. They also can't totally appreciate the pain and sacrifices we make to get to this point. Many of these people have a difficult time understanding why you just aren't happy and relaxed about being pregnant. These attitudes can be communicated in subtle ways that cause us to hide our true feelings. Sometimes, we stop talking to people, and they never know why. Don't cut people off because you are afraid to express your true feelings and fears. Usually, if you are open with people who support you, they will validate and help you.

In my interview with Sue and Howard we addressed her pregnancy. Sue said: "It was frightening and scary. Not a fun relief thing at all. Now what's going to go wrong? Now are we going to lose this pregnancy? We did have a lot of stuff going on our first trimester. We thought it was over—[that] kind of thing. " She continued: "Then I have the heightened fear that something would go wrong in the end, like in the delivery or that the baby would come out and be deformed. I am sure everybody has those fears, but I feel, for me, they were heightened."

Howard added: "I think you appreciate it a lot more. I think we appreciated every stage of pregnancy a lot more than somebody who just tried and got pregnant. Got pregnant and enjoyed it."

Sometimes, it's hard to ask for support. You and your spouse may also have a difficult time understanding why you just can't sit back and enjoy your pregnancy. If you tell family and friends, they may also be confused about this. You may find yourself experiencing feelings of guilt because you are not relishing the pregnancy you worked so hard to achieve. Those of us who have experienced an unsuccessful pregnancy or unsuccessful attempts at pregnancy will always feel some element of stress relating to subsequent pregnancies. This is normal and it is important for you to realize this. Don't isolate yourself because of guilt over these feelings.

Another thing that commonly leads us into isolation is the feeling we are "in between" the infertile and fertile worlds. We feel we have left behind the world of infertility, but we may still have a sense of loneliness and isolation in relation to fertile parents. Fertile couples are usually looking ahead with excitement and joy. You may feel that you have to temper your feelings around them, just as much as you would around your infertile friends. You really can't fully engage in either realm, so where can you go? Try to identify a friend or family member you can openly share your feelings with (both happy and sad). You need a full confidant in addition to your spouse. You may have things you won't want to say to your spouse, for a multitude of reasons, and you shouldn't carry them around. Allow yourself moments to complain to a trusted person about the times when you don't feeling well, either physically or emotionally. If you are in real need of regular support, then joining or forming a PAL group is a good idea. This is often the best way to be proactive about recognizing your needs and doing something about them.

There are also many little things you can do for yourself to alleviate the physical and emotional stress of pregnancy. Allow some time to pamper yourself. Take a warm bath. Do some deep breathing in a quiet, relaxing place. Light some candles. Do things you know will offer you some comfort and relax you. Exercise is an important stress reliever for many women, and yet some women who would never miss a day in the gym stop cold when they get pregnant. They fear exercise may endanger their pregnancy. But pregnancy is a challenging physical and psychological state. Regular, appropriate exercise can help with some of the aches and pains of pregnancy, relieve stress, and help you sleep better. Sleep problems are quite common in pregnancy, and they can compound emotional stress.

If you have any doubts about what things are safe or not while pregnant, be sure and consult your physician. For example, you may want to change your exercise routine to walking rather than running, or you should know that going into a Jacuzzi is often not recommended during your pregnancy. Sometimes, we can readily identify things we could do to make our pregnancies go more smoothly, but find it hard to create the time or the energy. Don't give up, though—seek support instead. Let your friends or family know what they can do to help you make those things happen. Sometimes we need a partner for those walks, or someone to stand in for our other obligations, so we can take needed time off. Think about how others could support you in your efforts, and then don't be afraid to ask them.

I shared Sue and Howard's fears during my pregnancy. My husband remained the eternal optimist. You just become used to having something go wrong, so you have a heightened sensitivity towards it, and almost begin to anticipate it in order to prepare yourself emotionally for what comes next. Every test and visit to the doctor becomes a milestone. I didn't actually believe I had a healthy baby until we delivered her and she looked at me and latched onto my nose.

Pregnancies that occur without any type of infertility treatment can cause difficulties such as weight gain, sleepless nights, pains in your back, swelling in your feet, and problems with nausea or eating. These problems are compounded when intertwined with the stress and anxiety experienced during your infertility treatment. There is often an underlying fear that there is some undetected medical problem related to symptoms that may ordinarily occur during a pregnancy.

Infertility treatment adds an additional layer of worry to a "normal" pregnancy. For example, during my pregnancy the doctor recommended I have amniocentesis. I had trepidations about having this procedure, because there was a small chance that my fetus could be injured during the test or that it would result in a miscarriage. After all the things we had gone through to get pregnant, I did not want to take a test with even a one percent chance of harming my baby. We ultimately opted for another test, a level-two ultrasound which gave my doctor the information she needed to confirm that my baby was developing normally. This test was not invasive in the same way the amniocentesis would have been, and it did not jeopardize my baby in any way.

Women have many anxieties during pregnancy. We had a friend who had a doctor suggest she go on bed rest to ensure that her pregnancy went smoothly. She had suffered from a number of miscarriages, and opted to put her work life and all other areas of her life on hold. She spent months on bed rest to ensure, as best she could, that she would have a normal pregnancy and a healthy baby. She ultimately did have a healthy baby boy. The quest to have a healthy baby remains strong throughout our pregnancy, and can be intensified when you experience infertility. When we need extensive infertility treatment to get pregnant, this can intensify our insecurities, and these worries will indeed influence decisions we make throughout our pregnancy.

Even in the labor stage of pregnancy, fears related to infertility treatment can arise in our thoughts and emotions. Before going into labor, my doctor accidentally nicked my placenta and broke my water during a routine examination. I immediately assumed something was wrong and I was going to lose my baby. Later, during hour sixteen of my labor, my doctor informed me that my baby was just not coming out, and I was not dilating and pushing as effectively as they had hoped. My doctor began talking about performing a caesarian section on me. Here I was, in the final minutes of my labor, and I remember flashing back to all of the infertility trials and tribulations we had gone through to get to this moment. I just wanted to do whatever my doctor told me to do to expedite a safe delivery. I prayed my baby would be healthy. Even in these last moments, I had to hold back old fears that something was going to go wrong, and my body would fail me and my baby. This is a common experience for new moms, and can be heightened by the infertility experience.

THE ONGOING ROLLER COASTER RIDE

One of the things infertility treatment does is heighten your awareness of your body. Believe it or not, this is intensified when you become pregnant. Every ache, pain, unexpected movement—or lack of movement—terrifies us. I remember getting a phone call from my obstetrician while I was at work. She told me I should feel my baby move every hour, and if I didn't notice any movement after an hour, I should come into the office right away. It was nearly impossible for me to work after that, because I just sat there waiting for my baby to move. It was over an hour before the next kick, and I was convinced something was wrong after the comment she had made. I was really frightened, just sitting there waiting for something to happen and feeling totally helpless.

The good news is that, as you get farther into your pregnancy, many people find the intensity of their anxiety often does begin to subside. You may find that your emotions still feel much like a "roller coaster" throughout your pregnancy, though. It helps to read and educate yourself regarding your body and the changes caused by pregnancy. Knowing what to expect can also help you to cope with any residual anxiety and fears. Make sure the doctor and nurse that are working with you are aware of your infertility history, so they will be more sensitive to any concerns or fears you may be expressing.

Several women I have worked with have talked about a particular example of this. They grew quite anxious between their ultrasounds, because the length of time felt long to them. Seeing an ultrasound and hearing the heartbeat of their baby was a way for them to feel certain their baby was safe and healthy. It was a source of real comfort for them. They related these fears and their histories to their doctors, and they came to an agreement where the women could come in for an ultrasound much more frequently, if they felt the need. This would never have happened if they had not shared their concerns and histories with their doctors. You too can come up with some workable plan to address your particular needs, if you are willing to sit down and discuss it with your doctor. It may mean that you are given permission to make more phone calls or have more frequent doctor appointments. Remember to write down the questions you want to ask or special requests you have before your doctor appointment.

Sometimes people feel it is more difficult to form a connection or a bond with their baby, because they are afraid of losing it. Your spouse may also experience more distance from your pregnancy as a defense mechanism. You need to be careful about not misinterpreting this reaction and perceiving it as a lack of support. You need to be able to openly discuss this issue with your partner. The first trimester may be a time when this occurs. This can sometimes also be an issue for people who have babies through a donor process or surrogacy. Often, people find that once the child is born this connection or bond does occur right away.

If this does not happen for you, you may want to seek counseling to explore what you can do to cope with this situation. There are many reasons that people may initially feel an emotional distance while pregnant. Most commonly, this reaction is a shield people put in place to protect themselves from the potential disappointment they would feel if they lost their child. It is a self-defense mechanism. Some husbands try to remain more detached, because they feel they may need to provide extra support for their wives in the event of a crisis during pregnancy. Staying detached is their way of preparing to deal with the worst. If this emotional distancing continues, however, particularly after the child is born, then it's a good idea to address these bonding issues through counseling.

Disclosure is another issue that can surface during pregnancy. Sometimes, we put off telling people about our treatment or the details of what we are doing. We think that if we don't get pregnant, there's no need for people to know. But now that we are pregnant, we have to decide what to tell people. If you haven't told people before, you need to give careful consideration to what information you are going to give to friends, your family, and, most importantly, to your eventual child. The things you disclose now will likely be known someday by your child, and you should give careful thought to what you want your child to know about how he or she was conceived. You should also think about how you would want them to find out.

You may decide to say nothing, but this is hard to do when you are pregnant. Think carefully about the timing of it, and decide in advance what and when to tell people about your pregnancy. Often, you will be telling your family, your friends, your acquaintances, and your employer. You may not tell them all the same thing, but sometimes it's good to tell a consistent story, even if the level of detail you go into varies. Make sure your partner and you are in agreement about these all-important questions, and that you both act consistently. I will be discussing disclosure in greater detail in Chapter 17, so you may want to review the information in that chapter very carefully before you decide how to handle these important decisions.

Once you decide about disclosure, you may still not be sure what to say. When we start telling people about our journey, they often ask questions, and the answers can be mystifying or technically hard to explain. In the first chapter of this book, I used a multitude of terms that are often associated with infertility. I specifically mentioned some with regard to treatments used by the people I interviewed. If the early chapters don't help you form the explanations you want, then there is a more comprehensive list of information that can be of value in the glossary in Chapter 21. Consulting the glossary may help you sort out what to say.

Infertility treatment is filled with terms and language that can be totally foreign to us and to others who have never been exposed to it before. The medical teams that work with us use these terms with total comfort on a daily basis, and sometimes need to be reminded when they use a word or initials that we are not familiar with. Don't be afraid to talk with your doctor or medical team about the exact nature of your treatment, even if this seems after-the-fact. Often, we are so absorbed with moving forward, that we put trust in our medical team and don't pay attention to all the details during treatment. Once you are pregnant, though, you should have a very clear understanding of what happened in your treatment. This is critical to deciding what to tell people and how to tell it. Naming a procedure can become disclosure, so be aware of this, and be sure you tell people exactly what you want them to know. Remember, one of your most important guides should be the disclosure you want your child to have in the future.

Whether we are aware of it or not, we do bring our infertility history with us into our pregnancy. The challenges that go along with that are great, and should be recognized. You also need to recognize that you will bring a variety of coping skills and the inner strengths you developed while on your journey. These skills and strengths were what helped to bring you to this unbelievable stage of pregnancy. You have doubtlessly experienced the roller coaster ride, but hopefully you have found ways to be empowered, too. This knowledge and these skills will help you face the challenges and find the joy that lies ahead as your pregnancy proceeds. We can't avoid the ups and downs, but we can recognize them for what they are and keep moving forward.

CHAPTER 14
PARENTING AFTER INFERTILITY

Those of us who have traveled down the path of infertility know all too well about the hardships associated with it. It is a trauma or crisis that occurs in our lives, and we are forever changed by it. If we are lucky enough to emerge into the role of parents, we take those feelings with us. It is important to step back and take some time to look at the effect our infertility has on us when we become parents. I believe taking the time to examine this will help us be better parents. When faced with infertility, we spend all our time and energy thinking and focusing on trying to conceive or adopt a healthy child. Then suddenly we are there, and we have to switch gears and think about the role of being a parent rather than an infertility patient.

Patricia Johnston addresses the issue of parenting after infertility (PAI) in her book, *Taking Charge of Infertility*. She discusses the impact of infertility on becoming a parent. She tells us: "Because a full-blown infertility experience has created such a difficult road to parenthood, it would be unrealistic to say that it doesn't have any effect on how you parent. Of course it does. Because of infertility you have faced a major life crisis, often much earlier than others of your peers. Infertility has tested your relationship with your partner and very likely affected your style of communication and the level of your intimacy. Because of infertility you have had to examine your motivations for parenthood upside down and inside out in order to justify spending enormous amounts of time and money and physical capacity and emotional energy in a quest either to conceive or to adopt. Infertility has very likely changed you in significant ways."(36)

I have spent a lot of time around people who have had children as a result of infertility treatment or adoption. One thing I have noticed is that they feel a strong incentive to gather as much information and education as they can. Parenting has been an important goal from the moment they began their infertility journey. Whether their children were adopted or they became parents through treatment, this group is strongly motivated to be good parents. There is an ongoing sense of amazement and gratitude around being given the opportunity to parent, and often this does not seem to go away. The other piece of this feeling is that, generally, the opportunity to parent is not taken lightly.

After I had my daughter, I became a member of a parenting after infertility (PAI) group. I really recommend this for a lot of reasons. You have an opportunity to meet other parents who have gone through what you have. We all speak the same language and have struggled with similar issues. So, if one of us is trying to decide what to do with those frozen embryos, we all understand immediately what the issues are. We also know that we are surrounded by people who understand and support us. Difficult issues can continue after you become parents. New issues like disclosure arise. It is very helpful to have a sounding board of fellow parents to talk with about how they are tackling these problems. Mostly, the moms meet in my group, but we do have occasional gatherings, where the dads can participate as well.

Early on in our PAI group, the members shared their feelings about becoming parents, and their stories were similar to those told by Sue and Howard. In our group, we have guest speakers, and we exchange resource information. We also make time to treat ourselves to a night out to relax. Sometimes that can be very hard to do when you are the parent of a small child. The other wonderful piece of our group is that it serves as a playgroup for all our kids. This is special because all of our kids are here as a result of infertility treatment. They will be growing up with other kids who were brought into this world in the same way. Down the road, it may be nice for them to have peers they can talk with and relate to about this. When the time is right to explore their origin questions and feelings, they will know others who have the same experience. They are all growing up together, so they know other families like their own, and it doesn't seem so rare. This provides a strong normalizing component to their view of these questions.

THE CHALLENGES OF PARENTHOOD

Being a new parent is one of the most challenging undertakings in life. Newborns are completely dependent and helpless. Crying is their only way of communicating needs. They can only eat a small amount and so they need to feed around the clock. As a new parent, you lose sleep and are shackled to your baby's care twenty-four hours a day without end. New moms have the added difficulties of recovering from delivery and weathering the hormonal upheavals of the end of pregnancy and the beginning of lactation. Some women experience bonding issues early on or even full blown postpartum depression. Breast feeding is often difficult to initiate, and this can be particularly true for older moms. Many new parents think that things like breast feeding and bonding will come naturally, and they are surprised when these take time and effort. All this is as true for new parents after infertility, as it is for others. Sometimes parenting after infertility intensifies these issues, and this can be particularly true in adoptions.

Yet, because people who have been through infertility treatment experience a lot of ups and downs, they often do not seem to be as overwhelmed by the ups and downs of parenting. I think one reason for this may be that the infertility journey requires you and your partner to have a lot of ongoing communication and creates a cooperative, team-like environment that can work well when you are the parents of children. I want to be clear that I do not mean to say that people who parent after infertility treatment are always better parents. That is not the case at all. I am just saying that the dynamics within a couple can change and be strengthened as a result of the infertility experience. Surviving the infertility experience can strengthen people's motivation to be good parents because they worked so hard to get there. You are forced to make difficult decisions quickly, be flexible, and cope with unexpected things while undergoing infertility treatment. Above all, you learn to support each other. These are skills that come in handy when you are parenting.

There is another dynamic at play for those of us who parent after infertility. When we face the common challenges of pregnancy and parenting, we frequently don't accept our feelings. We may have a very difficult pregnancy or labor. We may have a child that has colic or has a bad temper. We are not able to sleep. We are adjusting to our new baby. Maybe the bonding process doesn't go well at first. Your child may not sleep well, may be short-tempered, and may cry a lot.

There are times in every parent's life where there is a level of frustration and, at times, anger as well. With PAI parents there is an element of guilt that goes along with this. We waited so long and went through so much to have this child come into our families and into our lives, and then we become angry with the child. These feelings seem unacceptable.

We made reference to the bargaining phase many people go through, where we make promises about what we will do if we are lucky enough to have a child come into our lives. Then, we know we are not being the kind of parent we promised we would be. We say to ourselves, "I desperately wanted this child and I am not even doing a good job of taking care of my child." You may get angry at yourself or at the child. While you were going through the infertility treatment or the adoption process, you made silent promises to yourself and to the child you hoped would come. You promised to be a super parent. This is a promise that is not possible to keep. These feelings are normal. Every parent has moments of anger. Try to get a handle on the guilt and step back and think about why and where it is coming from. That will help you take control of some of those guilty feelings you may find yourself struggling with.

There also may be times where the child becomes a source of conflict between you and your partner. You may disagree on a parenting style. One of you may feel that the other is not doing his or her fair share. As the child gets older, there may be some splitting that occurs, where the child may play one parent against the other. Suddenly the relationship that you have with your partner has changed. Maybe one of you is jealous and feels that the other is giving to much attention to the child. This can be very confusing and disruptive for a couple that worked so well as a team going through the infertility journey together. Lots of mixed emotions can be stirred up and you may not know where to go with them.

Some of us assume that, when the child finally comes, everything will be all right and fall into place, because we deserve it after all we went through to become parents. When this doesn't happen or new conflicts rise up, it can be immobilizing and perplexing. Some of the dynamics that I described above can occur in many families. It is not unusual. It is just that our feelings are intensified as a result of our previous infertility experience. Our expectations about our parenting may be unrealistic. Try to maintain perspective and be realistic about what you are and aren't able to do as a parent. Remember what you said and did, how you communicated with your partner before the child came. Think about what made you an effective team. Try to reinstate some of these techniques if you can. It will help you feel like you are regaining control of the situation.

It is tough when everyone is sleep deprived and on edge. You may need to take some time for the two of you. I will address couples issues more in Chapter 19. You may need to consult a family member, trusted friend, or a therapist. Don't let these kinds of poor relationship dynamics go on too long without addressing them. Solo parenting can be a way of withdrawing from your partner. It seems self-justifying, because you have to focus on the baby's needs, but it also a common way that barriers and resentments are built up in relationships. The longer this goes on, the harder it is to stop. Also, the negative feelings that go along with this disruption in your family dynamic are compounded over time. They may then emerge in moments and in ways you don't want them to.

I remember when my daughter was born I really wanted to connect with other older parents who had young children. I wanted to have other people to talk to, who had something in common with me. I was totally naïve about how to go about finding these people. I went to local parks. I went to some day classes at my health club. I took lots of walks and sort of looked around for potential candidates. My search was not very successful. One day I struck up a conversation with a young girl, who couldn't have been more than 20. She had a young child. It was very apparent to me that we had very little in common. After that conversation I was aware that I was feeling an acute sense of isolation. It felt good to at least talk with somebody besides my husband. But I felt very out of place and I knew I would not feel comfortable talking to her about some of the issues unique to having a child as a result of infertility treatment.

Through RESOLVE, I later found out there was a group near me, and there were two other women who lived just a few blocks away.

Joining some type of group really does help you prevent that sense of isolation that can occur after bringing a child in your life. It's not always easy to find a peer group, but this is a very valuable thing to have as a new parent. It takes some energy to get out the door sometimes, but the rewards can make it worthwhile.

Patricia Johnston, in *Taking Charge of Infertility,* talks about how to overcome the feeling of being an inadequate parent. Her recommendation is to try to educate yourself as much as you can through books, classes, and workshops. I also think talking to people you trust and respect who are parents is very helpful. Use resources like your pediatrician, teachers, school counselors, or therapists. Parenting magazines can also help guide you through the parenting challenges you will surely face.

BUILDING HEALTHY FAMILY ENTITLEMENT

Ms. Johnston also looks at the critical issue of entitlement. This is an issue for parents in all families, regardless of how the family is built, but it is intensified by the infertility experience. Fundamentally, parents and children should feel they are entitled to mutual love and belonging. She quotes Dr. Jerome Smith on this subject. Dr Smith wrote a book about adoption, but his concepts are applicable to all people who are parenting after a struggle with infertility. Ms. Johnston says that Dr. Smith articulated "the need for parents and children to come to believe that they are entitled to and deserving of one another and that they belong together."(36)

A healthy sense of entitlement is important to the mutual sense of security around the parent-child relationship, particularly when parents need to impose limits on their children. Ms. Johnston goes on to say: "For those who do not feel a healthy sense of entitlement as parents discipline can be a problem. The inability to be gently but firmly consistent and to follow through with logical consequences, an unwillingness to be seen as a 'bad guy' for fear of losing the love of a child, or (in any variety of adoption) an unexpressed feeling that a genetic parent somewhere is more 'real' than are you and might not approve of your parenting, all are signs of an incomplete sense of entitlement."(37)

Ms. Johnston identifies a common, critical insecurity of parents, which can be amplified by parenting after infertility. If adoptive parents or parents who have their child as a result of infertility treatments are unable to come to terms with their entitlement fears, the end result can be an unhealthy parent-child relationship. This can be particularly true when the potential for unfair (and unrealistic) comparisons between themselves and the genetic parents exists. The lack of a strong sense of entitlement can tear a family apart, because it inhibits the ability to set healthy limits, have full communication, and build strong, trusting relationships. In this case, the family will become dysfunctional and, if this poor sense of entitlement is not addressed, the family will tend to stay dysfunctional.

Ms. Johnston discusses the recommendations that Dr. Smith makes to establish a stronger feeling of entitlement. They consist of three steps. The steps include the following: "...recognizing and dealing with feelings about infertility, recognizing and accepting the differences which are a part of adoption, and learning to handle reflections of the societal view that adoption is a second best alternative for all involved. Once pointed out, these issues for adoption built families are obvious, and it isn't too difficult for most to see how this particular aspect of adoption applies to those who have built quasi-adoptive families with the assistance of third parties. It's a little less clear why those who have given birth to a child genetically related to both of its social parents might feel less entitled to their children than do parents who have not gone through infertility."(38) Ms. Johnston points out that the infertility experience can impact the sense of entitlement for anyone who comes through this experience to parent afterward. This is important for all of us to recognize as we struggle to be good parents.

The infertility journey is difficult, and it changes us. Part of the challenge is dealing with some of the negative perceptions of society, particularly when we become parents. Society generally views genetic parents as "more justified" in the way they treat their children, and people can seem to extend greater trust to genetic parents. On the other hand, society can remain suspicious of non-genetic parents. These societal signals are things we internalize as we go through infertility treatment and afterwards. Social ambivalence compounds the feelings of insecurity that we often have throughout our infertility journey. Often these feelings begin with the loss of control we have over our bodies, and they can continue to plague us on some level as we become parents. But what parent doesn't feel a loss of control, in terms of their children, at some point in the child's development? It just may be a little more painful for those of us who are parents after infertility. That raw nerve is there. It is attached to those old feelings associated with the infertility journey, and the uneasiness we felt about ourselves, as though we were failing at some level. These feelings can return and we can feel guilty when we need to set healthy limits for our children.

Just know that the job description of being a parent, any parent, involves moments of self-doubt and uncertainty associated with raising your child. You can approach these moments head on by arming yourself with education and knowledge. Remind yourself that others go through it—other people who have not had infertility treatment. Nobody is the perfect parent, and nobody is the total expert on all aspects of parenting. Review the steps toward healthy entitlement described by Dr. Smith. Think about what you need to do to help yourself and your partner achieve these goals. You will need to really focus on good communication between you and your partner. You should also seek the input of other trusted friends and family members. Building a strong sense of entitlement may involve some teamwork. You can do it. You have the abilities and the skills. Think about the strengths you tapped into to survive the infertility journey and to get where you are. Use these strengths and the other guidelines discussed in this chapter to help yourself gain confidence about your ability to parent. Know that you will make mistakes and accept this. It is a very realistic expectation. This is a gift you can give yourself, and it will help you be a more effective parent.

GROWING WITH YOUR CHILD

Parenting isn't easy, and the challenge of it transforms us. Sometimes, remembering your struggles with infertility can be a source of empowerment for this new challenge. What are some of the strengths that come about as a result of being a parent after the infertility journey? Think about it. Sue described earlier how it helped her become a more assertive person. Greater flexibility is another strength you may have developed. Maybe, you can question things in a way you wouldn't before. Life takes on a different meaning, and you are more grateful for things you might ordinarily have taken for granted. In your work with doctors and nurses and other healthcare professionals, you may have learned that the experts do not have all the answers. You may find that you have a heightened sensitivity towards yourself and your needs and also towards others. Perhaps this has instilled a greater sense of empathy. Perhaps one of the by-products for you has been a greater sense of self-confidence or an elevated self-esteem.

The role of being a parent is one that can bring you unimaginable joy, as well as many daunting challenges. You may be surprised to find as your child grows, develops, and changes that the same thing happens to you. The challenges of parenting your newborn baby are different than the challenges of raising a toddler. The bonds and ties that you will develop as you nurse, hold, and watch your newborn change and grow will seem to strengthen. Each developmental stage of your child can begin to feel like the best time and the best age you will have with your child. Sometimes, you don't want them to change, to grow up. But, as many parents told me, it just keeps getting better. Suddenly your toddler becomes a little person, who walks, talks, and goes to the potty on their own! And you think: it can't get any better than this! But it does, and so it goes.

Each stage of child development and parent development will have its share of challenges and wonderment associated with it. There will be things you won't want to let go of, like nursing your baby, or holding your child in your arms, or your child's expression when Santa Claus has come. There can be a feeling of loss as these early days wane and end, becoming wonderful memories. Yet, your children will continue to grow and learn from you. They will become more engaged with the world around them, and develop more expressive, charming, and independent ways. At times, they will frustrate our expectations or mirror us back at ourselves and our world, exposing our foibles. They can be so infuriatingly "right" about us sometimes. The bonds will be tested and hopefully strengthened, as they grow with time. May the same be true for us as parents! It is really something to watch as your children grow and develop their own personalities and interact with the people and world around them. As parents, we get to relive this discovery of the world through them, and this experience can shape and change us with rediscovery, too!

CHAPTER 15
RAISING AN ONLY CHILD

In Chapter 1 I mentioned secondary infertility, which is when a person is able to have a child (or children) but is unable to do it again. For those of us who undergo infertility treatment, if we are lucky, we will have a child at the end of our treatment. Afterward, there may or may not be the option to try and have another child. For many, it is like secondary infertility. Some couples chose not to pursue further treatment because of the expense, the physical discomfort or the life disruption. Others recognize that they were lucky and may not have the best chance of repeating success. Many people who undergo infertility treatment successfully will fall into this category, and decide not try again. They will turn their attention instead to raising an only child. There are issues associated with raising an only child, and in this chapter we will take a close look at them.

Today approximately 30 percent of the families with children have only one child. There are a lot of reasons for this. We all know that women are waiting longer to have children and, because they start later, they ultimately may only be successful one time. Some people wait to have children because of financial reasons, or they choose to have a single child so their limited financial resources can be focused on developing the potential of a single child. Another contributing factor is the ever-increasing divorce rate. Divorce has become quite common, and this can disrupt the growth of families. Sometimes, a death of a partner leaves the remaining parent a widow or widower, and there can also be the unexpected death of a sibling, which leaves an only child. There are many reasons for the growth of one-child families today.

Obviously, infertility plays a big part in all of this, and many women are not as successful as they used to be at having a baby. They are starting later, and many women are also more focused on their careers. They often put time and energy into their professional life before they choose to start having a family. They get married later in life and get divorced more frequently. The ongoing stability of the majority of families in the United States seems to be questionable.

There are so many pressures and stresses on families today, that it is growing increasingly difficult for them to remain intact. Better access to birth control is another big reason that more people have only one child today. For many people, having a child is a conscious choice, and they are waiting for the right time in their lives. There are even some people who have only one child for philosophical reasons, because they believe our society is already overpopulated and they don't want to add more children to the planet.

For those of us who have taken the infertility journey, there can be other issues related to having an only child. We may feel some guilt, because due to medical reasons, financial reasons, age, or health reasons we may not be able to have any more children. We may want to have other children, may want our child to have a sibling, but then find we cannot make that happen. Adoption is always an option, but many people decide not to pursue adoption for a variety of reasons.

As parents, having an only child can be the source of a number of concerns. We do not want our only child to feel burdened later in life by having sole responsibility for our care as we grow old. We would rather our child had a sibling to share in parental caretaking later in life. For some people—and older parents in particular—this can be an important source of concern. There are other reasons we might want to have additional children. If we have had positive relationships with our siblings, we might want our child to experience this as well. You can't always assume that the sibling relationship is going to be a positive one (think about the current relationships of siblings you know). There are many people who are not close with their siblings or don't have a good relationship with them. Ongoing conflicts between siblings are fairly common, and it isn't a given that having another child will ensure a strong and positive sibling bond for your child. But it's rare for parents of only children not to think about the lack of siblings as a loss for their child.

Having additional children can also mean additional financial hardships on a family. It can also impact people's work and their careers. Having a second or third child does have an impact on your relationship with your oldest child. There may be issues of jealousy, competition, and anger that arise as a result of your need to share your attention with the new child. It can cause stress on a marriage if the addition of a child is not by mutual consent. Sometimes, trying to parent more that one child can cause unexpected conflict in a marriage. Time management and juggling the caretaker, parent, work, and spousal roles becomes more complicated and difficult. Talk to any parents with two small children, and they will tell you it is more than twice as hard as having only one.

Some people have preconceived ideas about only children, and believe they are being somehow developmentally damaged. Some people think that the personality or emotional development of only children is negatively affected by the lack of siblings in their lives. Research has proven this idea to be erroneous, and it has also revealed some surprising findings about only children. They tend to be more comfortable in their relationships with adults. This is partially due to the fact that only children tend to be around adults more, interacting with them on a more regular ongoing basis than children with siblings. Only children tend to be more achievement-oriented, and they use adults as role models, rather than older siblings. Only children tend to develop a greater sense of self-confidence, partly because people don't make the kinds of comparisons with them that are commonly made between siblings. They don't have to deal with the intense pecking order and rivalries that are often part of growing up with siblings. Only children get to be themselves and define their own world.

Only children can have other developmental advantages, too. In generally, families with one child have more financial resources available than families with multiple children. This means that an only child may have better educational opportunities available to them than the multiple children found in other families. Only children may have more early exposure to experiences and enriching activities because this is more affordable to their families. The same can hold true as they enter the school years. The parents of an only child often have more financial resources and time to devote to creating the best educational opportunities for their child.

PARENTING AN ONLY CHILD

As parents, when we have an only child, we have the luxury of showering them with all of the attention we can give. I believe that this is particularly true for kids who were conceived through infertility treatment or who were adopted. Their parents worked extremely hard and often made many sacrifices to become parents. They are especially invested in their kids, and generally do not take parenting for granted. Often, it was so difficult to bring these children into their lives, that these parents are willing to invest more time, effort, and attention to their children after they arrive. My experience with people who became parents after infertility is that they choose to spend as much time as possible with their kids, and they try to make it quality time. They are very invested in playing with their kids, helping them, and making meaningful contributions towards their education, growth, and development. They tend to be fully engaged.

I should emphasize again that I am not saying that other parents are not also invested in their children in similar ways. Whether you have children through infertility treatment or adoption or you don't, this won't necessarily change the kind of parent you are going to be. However, I do believe the infertility component has an impact on the nature and the dynamics of the relationships that develop between parents and children. It can help strengthen parental bonds and add another dimension to their family relationships.

There are some unique issues that arise in families with only one child, and I thought it would be helpful to take a look at some of them. They are not necessarily good or bad, but just things it is helpful for parents to be aware of and respond to. One very important thing that we do in our family is give our only child regular exposure to situations where she can interact with other children. From an early age, I have tried to give our daughter an opportunity to interact with other kids on a daily basis. This can be done in many ways. Just going to local parks or walking around your neighborhood is a good way to meet other kids and their families. This informal contact offers ongoing socialization for your child. Participating in a playgroup is an easy and inexpensive way to meet other kids. There may also be daycare, pre-school, or religious programs available for your child, which can give them both socialization and more formal learning opportunities.

The greatest advantage of daycare or pre-school programs is that your child can get used to separation from you. This can be a big issue for many only children, and a big issue for their parents, too! The tendency of some parents with only children is to always care for them and never entrust them to babysitters or daycare situations. This can be particularly true for people who have become parents after infertility. Some parents of only children dedicate themselves completely to their child's care, which is a necessary part of parenting a baby, but not a two year old. Be careful not to develop an unhealthy co-dependency with your child as he or she grows older.

It's natural for children to cry when they have their first separation experiences. The parents of only children will sometimes give into their own insecurities in these situations and not leave their child. Children are good at redirecting after you're gone, particularly if someone else is engaging them, but you have to leave. I introduced my daughter to separation by using the daycare at my health club. I was always close by, if she had a real meltdown, and the first separations were short in duration. She got familiar with the setting, and soon enough she was instantly ready to play without me around. Separation can be an issue for only children, and it's often good to give them early exposure to safe play situations without you there. Later, when she was two, I enrolled my daughter in a regular daycare a couple days a week for a longer period of time. She thrived on the socialization and by the time kindergarten rolled around, she was ready to go to the big school without any trepidation. Meanwhile, some of the other only children were having a real hard time separating from their mothers—and vice versa.

Strengthening the ties between you, your family, and your extended family is another way to create social opportunities for your child. Make a point of having the kids get together. Have pictures of cousins or other close friend's kids in your house and talk about them frequently. Try to spend time with them regularly and often, so that your child knows who they are and has the opportunity to develop an emotional bond with them. Cousins are a good way to expose only children to other kids of a variety of ages. Younger children are often interested in older kids, and vice versa. Sometimes, kids of different ages end up playing better together, or an only child can learn how to deal better with peers by observing how siblings of different ages interact.

One of the key techniques of good parenting is to have structure and rituals. Keeping regular hours for bedtime, mealtime, naps, and play is critical for children. Often, if left to themselves, kids will continue activities longer, put off eating and sleeping, and then end up crashing against a limit of hunger or fatigue. Sometimes it's hard to get them to transition, and the parents of only children can be particularly indulgent at times. This is where consistent rituals around bedtime and mealtime can make a big difference. Kids need signals that prepare them for what's next in their day. Reading books is an excellent transition to bedtime, for example, and if done as an everyday ritual will prepare your child instantly for sleep.

We have a special bedtime ritual with our daughter that she has responded very positively to. We sing a lullaby to her that my mother sang to me. My mother has been dead for many years, and singing this lullaby is a way for me to connect with my mother even though she is gone. It brings me comfort. A friend who observed us singing the lullaby was amazed at how my daughter immediately calmed down upon hearing the song. It is like a tonic to her. It also gives me a chance to talk to my daughter about her grandma, and this helps keep my mother's memory alive in a meaningful way for me, my daughter, and my husband.

There is another significant technique we use as part of our bedtime ritual. Every night, when we are getting ready to put her in bed, the last thing we do is talk with her about all of the people who love her. We start with Mama and Pa and then name grandparents, aunts, uncles, cousins, and close friends, including many she views as aunts and uncles. Sometimes she will name them. We then talk about what a lucky girl she is to have so many wonderful people in her life who love her. That's one of the last things she hears every night before she goes to bed. I do this because I believe it instills a strong sense of love and acceptance in our daughter. It reminds her how many people there are in her life, offering her unconditional love and support. It reminds her of family members who do not live close by, and so strengthens those relationships as well. It makes her smile and there is no better way to fall asleep than thinking about all the people in your life who love you. Be sure to develop calming rituals with your child, and if you can, make visualizing other people part of that process.

BEING AWARE OF POTENTIAL ISSUES

One of the dangers of parenting only children is that we can become overprotective. This can be particularly true for parents who have undergone infertility treatment and have an only child. We are terrified about anything happening to them, so we can tend to be very overprotective. I know I have been guilty of this at times. We may approach our children as if they are very fragile, and not let them experience things all children should experience. We need to be cognizant of this and have an internal mechanism inside of us reminding us when this is occurring. This type of behavior can foster an unhealthy dependence that will impact the child in a negative way as they grow up. It can also negatively impact the child's sense of self-esteem and self-confidence. If a child doesn't have a chance to try new things and experience success, this can lead to negative repercussions.

All young children have a problem with sharing. I believe this is especially true for only children. They don't have the opportunity to share like children with siblings do, so it can become particularly difficult for them to share with other children and other people. I attended a parenting lecture given by a psychologist who specializes in working with families and children, and she used a wonderful metaphor that enlightened me about the concept of sharing from a child's perspective. She asked us adults to imagine a total stranger coming in our house, uninvited, and marching up the stairs to our bedroom closet. She then asked us to imagine that person, without asking permission, picking out our favorite dress putting it on and wearing it. As an adult how would this make you feel? Now think about how tough it is for a child to grasp the concept of sharing, and be okay with another child grabbing his or her favorite toy. Her message has stayed with me. If I know there are kids coming over, I may take my daughter's favorite toys and tuck them away, out of sight, to avoid potential conflicts and battles. But at the same time, I want her to know she will be expected to share her other toys with guests.

My daughter and I have made a little game of sharing, and my hope is that this will make the concept more comfortable for her. For example, if we are eating I will make a point of sharing bites of my fruit with her, and she will share bites of her potato with me. I remind her that this way we both get to have some fruit and potato, and I point out how nice that is. Our friends and families were wonderful about donating clothes to us when our daughter was born. I always make a point of talking with her about that, when she begins to wear some of the hand-me-down clothing. I also believe in "clothing karma," and pass her toys and clothes on to friends and family. Then I try to point that out to her, when appropriate, so she has a sense of sharing with others as they have shared with her. When she is playing with other children and they let her use their toys, I always praise them, and I praise her when she shares with them. Repeating this message frequently will instill its value in your child. Remember, these lessons will take time to sink in, because it is just not natural for a young child to willingly share, but hopefully your child will eventually take on this value.

One downside of being a parent with an only child is that you don't have anything to gauge the child's accomplishments against. You can't compare your child's growth and development to another sibling. One tendency can be to sometimes go overboard when your child does achieve something, because to you it seems like a big deal. Another tendency can be to let your child fall behind normal developmental stages because you are not aware of what is age appropriate. Kids, of course, develop at different rates, and we shouldn't get overly excited or disappointed by their "accomplishments." We should be aware of developmental stages, though, and what is appropriate for a given age. Pediatricians often provide us with this information, and it falls to the parents to gauge and facilitate appropriate development. This is particularly true for only children, who don't have siblings to emulate.

I have a great example of these dynamics from my life. The first time my daughter used her potty, my husband and I really played it up. We kept praising her and did a sort of a potty dance in the bathroom thinking it would make her feel happy and proud of her accomplishment. Well, that really backfired—we went overboard. It freaked her out and she ran out of the bathroom screaming, "No, I didn't do a good job." She wouldn't use her potty again for a couple of weeks. I became more matter-of-fact about it, and that was much more successful. I did notice that when my daughter was around other kids who were older and potty-trained, she was inspired to use the potty without any prodding from my husband or me. The message my young daughter so aptly taught us, was that those of us with only children should reward or criticize them on the appropriate scale. The story also illustrates the value of giving your child the opportunity to observe and model the behavior of other kids.

Children are great teachers, and they are also great communicators. I learned that as both a social worker and a parent. If we take the time to listen to them, they will tell us exactly what they want and what they need. They have not learned adult tricks, like using indirect communication or hiding what they really think or feel. Only children can be particularly articulate sometimes, because they spend a lot of time one-on-one with adults. They can say what they mean and are often less intimidated about talking with adults. All children are incredibly honest. That was one reason I enjoyed working with them so much. What you see is what you get. Of course there is a downside to that. Sometimes your child will say something in front of somebody that is true, but you wished they hadn't said it. These are always special moments, and only children can tend to have more of them than most.

There is one other dynamic of the only child that I am painfully aware of as a social worker and a mother. In families with two parents and a single child, there is one guaranteed danger: the child will play one parent against the other. We are all aware of the case where a child asks for something, the mother says no, and then the child goes to the father, asks again, and the father says yes. I know I did that as a child. We all did. It seems that only children get particularly good at this technique, among others. Their ability to play us off against each other can ultimately cause a lot of conflict between their parents. Who has the power in this situation? Your child does, of course. That is not a good thing for any of you.

We were amazed as my daughter starting to try to play these games as early as the age of two. How do you handle this? The first thing to do is to be aware of what's happening, and the second thing is to make a point of keeping up strong communication between the parents. Check with each other about what is all right and what is not. Be sure and send your only child consistent messages from both parents. You can even do this regularly by communicating in front of the child. Don't undermine the authority of your partner, and make a point of correcting yourself, if you find you've been fooled into it. As your child grows older, if they know the two of you are going to talk about these things, it will tend to put an end to this type of behavior. You want to start doing this at a young age, so that these communication patterns are established. You also need to give your child the message that, if mom has said no to something, then dad will also say no.

There are lots of wonderful parenting books out there that can serve as great guidelines and tools for you. Talking with your friends and families is also a good way to get ideas. Many times, they know you and your child well, and you can get good advice from them about how to confront these situations as they arise. Parenting is always challenging, however you come to it, and however many kids you have. It never hurts to take advantage of the experience and wisdom around you. Raising an only child can have its special challenges, and I believe that some people tend to have negative perceptions about those raised as only children. A common stereotype is that they end up overprotected, spoiled, and selfish—something that can happen to all kids if their parents are fearful or thoughtless. I hope these parenting areas that I have discussed illustrate both the challenges and the positive opportunities of raising an only child. These children, like all children, can become very special, engaging, and generous people. This is especially true if you have fun parenting. Remember, even one child is a license to play, and playing well is one of the best lessons in life!

CHAPTER 16
MULTIPLE BIRTHS

When you hear about infertility treatment one of the common topics that comes up is the issue of multiple births. It is not uncommon to hear of a person having twins or even triplets after undergoing infertility treatment. The medications we are given have an impact on our fertility. Certain medications like Pergonal and Clomiphene can increase the chances of multiple births. Also when eggs or embryos are implanted it can directly affect the number of babies that a woman can ultimately have since multiple ova are used. It is not unusual from two or three eggs or embryos to be retrieved and implanted. This is done to try to optimize the possibility that a woman will get pregnant. For example, when three embryos are implanted in a woman's uterus, maybe one will not result in a pregnancy but two can turn into a successful pregnancy and ultimately result in the live birth of twins. I had three embryos implanted when I had my infertility treatment. When women are older, say in their forties, doctors are generally reluctant to use more than two embryos or eggs because they are concerned about the effect carrying and having multiple babies may have throughout the woman's pregnancy and during her labor. It can take its toll on our bodies and create additional health risks for the mother and the children .

The challenges of multiple births are interesting to say the least. Obviously it begins during pregnancy. Your abdomen will grow larger and you will be carrying more weight around than with a single birth. Sometimes multiple births may make normal pregnancy symptoms like nausea or swelling worse. Your doctor will detect more than one heartbeat during your examinations. You will need to see your doctor more frequently if it is determined that you are having more than one baby. The doctor will be monitoring you closely for any signs of medical problems or complications. Your nutrition also is especially critical in this situation. One of the problems associated with multiple pregnancies is early delivery and low birth rate. Good nutrition helps tackle the problem of low birth rate. You need especially good guidance in this area. You need more rest because the fact you are carrying more than one child takes more of a toll on your body. Another consideration is that the vitamins that you take must be adjusted to account for multiple fetuses. The information regarding the proper levels of care for yourself and your babies should be thoroughly discussed with your doctor, nurse, and midwife if you have one.

Some people may decide they are not able to take care of more than one or two children. There may be health risks or problems that necessitate considering doing a reduction. A reduction is when your doctor does a medical procedure to terminate one or more pregnancy in the case of multiple births. It is not a decision that is made lightly. There may be strong religious or ethical issues that you will struggle with in relation to facing this type of situation. This decision requires extensive consultation and discussion with your doctor and you and your partner to ensure you all understand the reason a reduction is being considered and you are all in agreement about how to proceed. Your doctor should outline the reasons the reduction recommendation is being made and the potential medical impact on you and all of the fetuses.

Obviously the delivery will also be affected by the birth of more than one baby. You want to be sure that you have discussed a labor and delivery plan with your doctor, midwife, and doula if you choose to have one. Make sure you all understand and agree with the components of this plan. Find out what medical treatment adjustments your doctor will be making in light of your multiple births. It may mean an earlier delivery. It may mean more bed rest for you prior to your delivery to ensure your good health and the health of your babies. There may be a longer labor and delivery. The medical team may need additional staff or equipment depending on how many babies your are having. Those of you who may want a home birth need to look carefully at what specific medical challenges the birth of multiple babies may offer to ensure that you have all of the appropriate medical attention you need at the time of your labor and delivery. Many healthcare professionals would recommend that you have your delivery done in a medical facility. Depending on how and when your delivery occurs, you and your babies may need to stay in the hospital for a longer period of time to ensure all of you are in good health. If the babies are born prematurely they may need assistance with taking in nutrition and breathing. Your doctor will want to be sure your babies are thriving and gaining weight before they are discharged. The good news is that the current medical treatment and technology available for babies in hospital neo-natal units is expanding. The survival rates for babies that are born weighing as little as two pounds has been steadily increasing. If your babies are born with a low birth rate and with some of the complications I mentioned above it is probable that they will have to stay in the hospital longer and you may be discharged without being able to take them home with you. This can be a very difficult and stressful time for new parents. You will be asked to continue to come to the hospital to spend time with the babies, to learn from the nurses and doctors about any special medical needs the babies might have. You will be asked to participate in their care and feeding using the guidance and support of the medical staff, midwife, and doula you have worked with.

The logistical challenges really emerge when you bring your babies home. Even though we all dream about the day we will bring our children home, it can be a particularly anxious time in the case of multiple babies. There is a big difference between a team of professionals helping you to take care of your children and you and your partner suddenly having to meet all of their care needs at home without instant consultation with a healthcare professional available. Especially in the case of multiple births you really want to make sure you have professional help like nurses set up to help you ease their transition home. These professionals will help you understand the challenges and demands you will be facing and the best way to meet these challenges. When we think about getting pregnant back at the early stages of infertility treatment we don't necessarily think in terms of having to get two or three cribs, strollers that hold more than one baby, multiple car seats, and clothing. Normal functions like feeding and changing diapers take on a whole new meaning when you have two or three babies crying. Teamwork is key in terms of facing these challenges. You and your partner need to really work together to develop a system that is workable. This could be a time when family and friends can also be called upon to assist you. Some people who have several babies have told me making a chart to keep track of feedings, naps, and diaper changes can be very useful as you begin to get to know your babies and what their needs are. There are organizations available that offer information, resources, and link you with other parents of multiple births. An example of this is the National Organization of Twins Clubs. They can be reached at 1-877-540-2200 or 1-248-231-4480. Your local chapter of RESOLVE would be able to link you with a member who also has more than one baby and they can clue you in about local support groups. It really helps to talk with somebody else who is tackling the parenting of multiples to get the additional insight and experience to help you figure out what will work for you and your family.

A member in our playgroup has triplets that are a month older than my daughter. When her kids were a year or so she would place a call to us when she was getting close to the playgroup site and a team of us mothers would go down to help her with transporting the kids, diaper bags, and clothes she needed to carry with her when she left her home. Just getting her kids dressed and fed was a huge challenge that could take all morning. The mothers in our playgroup were in awe of her patience and sense of humor. She had to really plan to take the extra time she needed to get her kids dressed and ready for the day. Once she was at the airport and one child ran in one direction and the other ran another way. She was traveling alone at the time. This was one example of the challenges she faced. She ultimately realized that if she was going out alone with them they would either need to be in a confined place like a playground with a fence, or she needed to have them on a leash-type of mechanism to keep track of them if they were in an airport.

The financial challenges are also an important consideration when you have multiple births. You may need two or three or more of everything needed to take care of a baby. That's lots of diapers, bottles, clothes, changing tables, cribs. Food costs are higher. Educational costs can be enormous.

The day-to-day challenges can be met if you are very

organized with the right amount of support—either professional, like a nurse or nurse's aid, family, or friends. Finding a babysitter or day-care can also be more difficult in this situation.

The rewards can be great as well. Your children can grow up and be very close. A friend who has twins told me that as her girls grew up they would speak to each other in their own secret language and finish sentences for each other. Their personalities were very different as well which she found interesting since they were identical. Some people prefer to only have to go through one pregnancy, labor, and delivery. They feel strongly that they want to have more than one child.

Being the parent of multiples offers its own unique challenges. There are more of these parents now than ever before. Parenting multiple children requires extra patience, money, flexibility, and strong organizational skills. A good sense of humor doesn't hurt either. It is critical for parents of multiples to work as a team as they approach the childcare and parenting responsibilities that lay ahead of them. Be realistic about what you can and can't do. Try as much as possible to treat each child as an individual with his or her own unique personality and needs. If possible, spending some individual time with your children is also important in terms of developing your relationship with them and helping enforce their individuality.

Finally, making time for work, for yourself, your marriage, and your relationship as a couple is extremely important. I realize it is also very difficult. It is hard to imagine having the strength to do this when you are at the end of a day when you were taking care of two-year--old triplets. Great daycare options certainly can help. Do what you can to make it possible. Look at the chapter "Becoming a Couple Again", for some marriage and relationship suggestions. There may be family members you can rely on to offer you some relief. Some places like Gymboree or local community classes, where you can leave the kids for a few hours with trained staff in a safe environment, may be a possibility for you. You need to try to make time so you can have a quiet dinner or see a movie. Maintaining this type of balance in your life may be one of the biggest challenges of all. Building the right support network can make this appear to be more of a reachable goal. The needs of your children will change as they grow and develop. Your needs may change with theirs. Include fun activities in your game plan. It will be helpful to you all as you face the days ahead as a family.

CHAPTER 17
DISCLOSURE

In earlier chapters I made reference to my belief that disclosure is one of the most difficult issues that people must struggle with as they go through infertility. In this chapter, I want to spend some time taking a look at how this relates to what we will tell the children who are here as a result of infertility treatment, surrogacy, or adoption. I want to repeat what I said previously, because it is critical to emphasize it: what other people know about how your child was born or came to you will probably be revealed to your child in the future. When considering disclosure, you need to remember this. Think about what you would want to tell your child about their origins, and when you would do this and how. Remember, when somebody else knows the story of your child's origins and you delay disclosure, there is always the possibility your child will learn the story from somebody other than you.

My husband and I were at a RESOLVE meeting in a small group, where this man told a story that brings this point home. He talked about growing up with his best friend for many years. They were adults. One day he overheard somebody talking about his friend being adopted. He went to his friend to ask him why he never told him about it. His friend didn't know what he was talking about. His friend went to his mother to ask her about it, and she confessed that he had been adopted and didn't know how to tell him. It was very difficult for him. He was very angry at his family for keeping this all-important secret from him. His parents never thought he would find out. That story has always stayed with me. It had a big impact on me. I promised myself that if we ever had a child there would be no secrets and we would share our story about how she or he became a part of our lives. The big question in my mind was how do we go about doing that?

I asked the people I interviewed about the issue of disclosure. Sue told me: "The funny thing about disclosure is we thought about it a lot while we were pregnant and when he was really little, and now it has kind of faded a little. It's to the point now where it is high on my list of things to do. I have to get this little book together and start to talk to him about it as much as I can. The normal parenting stuff is too time-consuming." I asked Sue what she and Howard had decided to do as a means of telling their son about how he came into their lives. They had given it a lot of thought. She said, "I wanted to start with him at age two. I always thought that I would have a little storybook for him because he can always understand a story. I want to make it in a format that would be appealing for him, which is a challenge. I have the book itself. It is a photo album that has like nursery rhyme type pictures. I have told him the story right before he goes to sleep while he is on my lap. I think I have the language down. The more pictures I can incorporate the more it will help him."

Howard added: "We almost have the video done. Now…I know him and know what he loves. I use the words 'gift lady' to describe the egg donor. One of the things I struggle with…is I don't want the story to begin with mommy and daddy. That's what we want it to be about—a mommy and a daddy. I have been struggling with: what do I want to call us, the husband and wife or use our names? Then we would tell him, one day we went to the hospital; and the baby that was there in the wife's tummy; came out, and that was you. That was the most wonderful moment of our life because that was you. It's just the before and what to call us." I was impressed with the amount of time and thoughtful consideration Howard and Sue had given to the delicate issue of disclosure. Their ideas about putting together some age-specific information for their son seemed like excellent advice. Their use of the term "gift lady" seemed like a very good idea that worked well for them and their son. Two good books that can help parents tackle these issues are *The Flight of the Stork: What Children Think (And When) about Sex and Family Building* by Anne Bernstein and *Lethal Secrets* by Annette Baran and Reuben Panor.

DISCLOSING TO A CHILD

You obviously have two choices about disclosure. You can choose to tell your child about his or her origins or you can choose not to. You need to look deeply into your heart and decide the reasons you are choosing to tell or not tell your child the truth about his or her beginnings. You need to balance the issue of privacy versus the issue of secrecy. For example, you may want to enable your child to have future privacy around these issues, but creating this in the future may require some secrecy now. This would probably mean keeping the secret from your child, too, until they know how to keep it themselves. You may feel that all this is too much of a burden to put on your child, or you may want privacy yourself around these issues. But you should think carefully about the balance between secrecy and privacy and its potential impact on your child. For example, does your child have a right to know about his or her medical history? In thinking about this, ask yourself if you would want to know about your genetic origins if you were conceived in this way. Why or why not? This is a very personal decision and you need to do what feels right for you.

My husband and I were in total agreement about telling our child everything about how she was born. We saved every piece of information we got, from the moment we began our infertility treatment. We plan on showing it to her, when she is ready. At the age of two, I started talking with her about her growing in my uterus. She is intrigued by these stories about when she was a baby and wants us to continue to tell them to her. She asks us to repeat them over and over in detail. What parent doesn't want to share the joyous story of having their child come into their life? That joy is infectious with your child. Then, at around age two-and-a-half, I began to tell her how I had trouble making a baby, and that we had to go to the doctor and get help from a special gift lady. We all need to figure out who we are and where we came from. Sharing information with our children about their origins during childhood can help them begin to put these pieces together for themselves.

I have been a member of a "Parenting after Infertility" group for over a year and a half now. Without exception, every mom in our group has talked about disclosure as a huge issue for her, and we all express some uncertainty and anxiety about where to go with it. That's one of the great things about this type of group. You can feel comfortable talking about issues like disclosure. I looked at these groups in Chapter 14. It is important to remember that disclosure is an ongoing process. You don't tell your child once and move on. The story of the origins of your child will change and become more detailed, as your child grows and wants more information. And your child will want more information. Your child will pick up cues from you about how to react to this information by how you give or withhold it. It is very important that you present the information in an age-appropriate way. Sue and Howard's story of a picture book and video for their young son is a great example of this.

I have often wondered what it is about giving our children this information that creates such anxiety for us. Is there a stigma to infertility treatment that we are afraid will be passed on to our children? Are we worried that once they learn the truth about their origins, they will harbor anger towards us? Maybe, we harbor fears that our children will reject us. Perhaps, we are concerned that having this information will somehow alter our child's self-esteem or feeling of belonging. Will our child think less of us for being unable to create a healthy child without the benefit of science and technology? I think that, on some level, it is possible that our own insecurities about our infertility get stirred up when we think about sharing this information with our children. Maybe, we worry that disclosure will undermine the development of a healthy sense of entitlement in our family.

Any or all of these issues may strike a chord with you. There may be other things that you can identify that cause anxiety when they are talked about in an open and honest fashion. Think about all of the jokes people make when they have to start talking with their kids about sex. The information you will be giving your child about your infertility journey can feel much more difficult and complex to convey. You may need to confront your own feelings about sex and your infertility.

My work as a social worker has given me the opportunity to work with many kids and their families. One thing I have learned is, if you do keep a secret from children, particularly adolescents, and they find out about it, they will feel a sense of anger. Trust will become a huge issue between you. If trust is destroyed, this can cause a functional relationship to turn into a dysfunctional relationship. An omission of pertinent information will be perceived by your child as a lie. You can ultimately rock the foundation of your child's world if you keep a secret like this from him or her, and then they discover this information from somebody else. The damage can be irreparable. Your child will start wondering what other information you have hidden from him or her. They will have doubts about your honesty from that moment on. This is particularly true for kids who are ten years old throughout adolescence. This period can be such a confusing time for them, anyway. If your child can't trust you, it will be difficult for a strong, lasting bond between you to be established and continue to grow. The child will feel betrayed.

Keeping the secret to yourself can also be a burden. Usually, some one else knows, even if it's only your partner. The burden of holding onto a secret can increase with time, and impact your relationships. Your or your partner's need to be relieved of the burden can be reinforced by the difficulty of disclosure. Waiting can make telling more and more difficult, because now the revelation may carry greater weight. The stakes may seem incredibly high. Disclosure could lead to surprise, hurt, and ruptures in your relationships. And yet, the burden you or your partner carry may seem to get heavier and heavier. Withholding information can snowball, as one omission leads to another, until the lack of disclosure seems to add up through the string of little lies you are forced tell. Eventually, this burden of withholding the truth can seriously impact your relationships, even if you manage to keep the secret.

If you do share information with your child about his or her origins, you want to ask yourself where he or she will go with this information. Will they understand it? Who will they share it with? Can they think about their own privacy, and will they be able to preserve it? Will your child want more information? Will the door be open for them to come back for follow-up information? You can be fairly sure that, as time goes on, there will be attempts from your child to get additional information. More questions will arise as they have time to think and digest the information that you share with them.

If for some reason you are not comfortable sharing this information with your child, there are other options for you. Again, this is a way for you to regain some control of the aspects of your life that infertility altered. You can have your partner, or a trusted friend or relative, be with you when you have this discussion with your child. Your partner or another trusted relative can talk to your child with the idea that you would be brought into the conversation at a later date. You should tell the pediatrician about your child's history, because there may be medical issues that arise where this information may be crucial. Remember, if you are not the one disseminating this information, the underlying message to your child may be one of shame or discomfort around his or her origins.

I believe the earlier you approach the topic of disclosure with your child the easier it might be. The reason for this is that there is a normalizing element to it, when it is presented at an early age, and when it is presented over and over again. The child will begin to get comfortable with it, if it is done carefully. Again the information you give must be age-appropriate, with understandable language and concepts used. Take some time before you have this discussion to think about what you are going to say. You may want to practice it with your partner or a friend or relative. Ask your doctor or a counselor about the approach you are using.

THE REACTIONS OF CHILDREN

I recently attended a conference that had a panel of four young women, ages fifteen to twenty-four. One was adopted, one the result of IVF, one had been a surrogate baby, and the other was a sperm donor baby. One of them accidentally found out at age nineteen how she was conceived, when an uncle made a comment, assuming she had known. It took her a year to work through the mixture of feelings she had. It was fascinating to listen to their perspectives. They universally agreed that parents should tell their children about how they were conceived. They also universally agreed that the timing should vary with the individual child and family.

One of the panel members was told when she was four. Another was told when she got sex education in high school. They all remembered when and how they were told. Each panel member said the most important thing a parent could do was to continue to let their child know that they love them. The panelists did not feel that the circumstances of their birth made them feel different or unusual in any way. They all chose to tell some friends, and none of them reported any negative consequences for discussing this with family or friends. It really solidified the concepts I discussed in the previous chapters.

There are a few things you want to keep in mind if you choose to disclose your child's origins to them. The first thing to remember is that you want to always tell the truth. You need to be honest. If you are not honest there is an underlying message of shame. Tell your child about his or her story in as simple a way as possible. You need to use language that your child will be able to understand. You may want to use some of the books that are already out there to help you with this. RESOLVE or a local bookstore can offer you advice about age and content-appropriate books for educating your child.

I mentioned earlier that disclosure is an ongoing process. You will be telling your child about their genetic origins on an evolving basis, which is contingent on your child's developmental stage. There are universal ideas that you want to focus on, as this story of your child's beginnings unfolds. If you incorporate these themes into the disclosure story, the chances of your child understanding and accepting this information will be greater. You must include an element of education around reproduction using the correct language. I will explain this in more detail a little later, but in general, you should use the correct terminology like sperm, and uterus, so as not to confuse your child as he or she gets older. Next emphasize that all families are special and unique, and that they are created in many different ways. Remind your child again and again that he or she is special, and you are very grateful that this child is a part of your life and your family.

You may want to use examples of other families to illustrate how different families can be. The family next door may have three boys and a girl, and can illustrate different size families or combinations of gender. Or, if you know families of a particular ethnic background, you could say, for example, "Robert's family originally came from a place called Mexico." Emphasize your ongoing feelings of uniqueness and unconditional love for your child. Finally, share with them the story about how they came to be your child in your family. As the child gets older you may want to share the decision process you went through, and talk about the type of infertility treatment you chose to have. If this involves a donor or surrogacy situation, then your child will likely want to know how you chose your surrogate or donor.

If you do decide to tell your child at a relatively young age, say a two- or three-year-old, one thing you need to keep in mind is the developmental stage of that child. Children at that young age tend to be very concrete in their thinking. They have a limited sense of abstract reasoning. Your goal is to normalize the way they were born. It is okay to use the correct terminology. Use words like uterus, embryo, or sperm when you are talking with them. You can choose to have a picture of the reproductive system with you and point to the correct parts of your reproductive organs as you tell your story. Pictures are a way to help young children learn and it is a good reference point for them. Explain that all babies are born when an egg and a sperm come together, and they become an embryo and grow in a woman's uterus. Explain to your child that all babies are wonderfully special and have their own unique qualities.

If you were involved in a donor or surrogacy situation, you need to tell your child that you were unable to get pregnant or make a baby without the help of your doctor and the gift of a wonderful person that helped create them. You should share that the donor or surrogate helped make them the person they are today. As your child gets older, you have to decide what additional information you want to give them about the donor or surrogate. Your child will want to know what the donor or surrogate looked like, and if you know them, and what kind of person they are. Older kids may ask you about how you found the donor or surrogate, and they may ask if you have a picture of them. Try not to take this personally. It is not a rejection of you. It is an attempt by your child to make some sense out of his or her origins, and their connection to his or her present world.

You may have limited information about your donor or surrogate. In the case of adoption, parental records may be closed. In many cases, your access to more information is limited at the beginning of the process, and these limitations will apply to your child, too. If you have more information or can get access to it, then you should think about how to explore this with your child. They will likely be interested, but you should both be ready to explore this together. Any time your child is not interested, don't push more information on them, but let them know it is there and can be explored when they are ready. If there isn't more information, then let them know this, too. In the absence of more of a story, you may want to explain how you chose the donor you did. You can talk about what special traits they had that you were hopeful would be passed on to your child. You can also discuss your beliefs around the role of nature vs. nurture in shaping us. This type of information can be helpful for your child to know, and sometimes leads to very fruitful origin discussions.

Remember many clinics and agencies currently continue to maintain a policy protecting the privacy and the identity of their donors. There are clinics and agencies you can go to where you are able to learn the identity or see a picture of the donor. Clearly, if the donor is a friend or relative they will be known. This situation needs to be handled especially carefully, so as not to confuse the child. In transparent situations, the parents and the donor need to spend a lot of time thinking about what messages the child will be given about how they were conceived and raised. When the child will have ongoing contact with the donor, a lot of time should be spent determining the role the donor will play in that child's life. There needs to be a clear agreement that can be consistently followed by everyone.

This issue was also addressed for the realm of adoption in Chapter 9. You need to determine ahead of time what kind of adoption you will be doing. If it is an open adoption, then clearly the biological parent may want to play a role in the child's life. How will that role be shaped? In the case of adoption or a known donor, there must be a consistent message given to the child regarding the involvement of the genetic parent. This message must be reinforced by all parties, so there is no confusion and no conflicting messages are delivered to the child. This dynamic will greatly impact how the child reacts to this information.

If you decide to disclose to your child, when should you do it? There is no correct answer to this question. You know your child better than anybody else. You know what they can handle, and what they can't. Young children are completely egocentric. They see the world as if it revolving around them and their needs. Their thinking is very concrete. They are looking for immediate gratification. They don't have a sense of the passage of time. They benefit from repetition. The advantage of starting earlier is that it is easier for you to tell the story. It can start out being quite simple. Also, if you tell it early on, then it becomes a part of your child's identity. It feels—and becomes—a very normal part of all your lives. It also gives your child a chance to integrate this information into his or her identity. The one thing to remember about starting with really young kids is that they won't get exactly what you are telling them at first. At an early age, they obviously don't have the cognitive tools to understand everything. Again, just be simple and consistent in your explanations. For example, Mommy wasn't able to produce the eggs that were needed to create a baby.

In the middle years of childhood, kids are at a cognitively higher level. These children will ask you more questions and demand more information and details about what you are explaining. Their abstract thinking is on a little higher level, but you should remember that it is far from fully developed at this stage. They may try to fill in the blanks with fantasy thinking in their own minds. Be sure and check back with them, and have them tell the story back to you. This is the best way to make sure they have a decent understanding about what you have told them. Your child may want to talk more about their origins at this age than they have in the past. You should be prepared to take the time and talk to them about this information. Once again, don't push them to explore this if they don't want to, but help them learn what they do want to know. Give them the space and time they feel is necessary to investigate their origins or to leave the subject alone.

As I said earlier, the adolescent years are not the best time to break this information to your child. It is a time of life where there is an ongoing struggle to fit in with peers and not be different. Kids this age are struggling to find their identities. They are also struggling for their independence, and trying to sort out how this struggle for independence will be juxtaposed with the reliance they have built on their parents. Many of us can probably remember what a hard time that was. There are all kinds of separation issues at this time of life, and raising the issue of infertility during adolescence can cause lots of uncertainty and confusion.

TRUSTING YOUR CHILD

I was in the middle of writing this chapter, when, by coincidence, RESOLVE was offering a seminar on disclosure, which I attended. There was a panel discussing issues around disclosure. One of the members of the panel was a fifteen-year-old girl who had been born through a surrogate. Her mother was in the audience as well. I was struck by her poise and wisdom, which was far beyond her years. Her mother spoke about the fact that fifteen years ago people didn't openly talk about surrogacy, because it was so new and not many people had done it. They were pioneers. Everyone in the room listened carefully to the personal story this girl told about her experience learning her birth origins.

This was my first opportunity to hear a reaction from the child's point of view. In this case she was not a child, but an adolescent. The message she gave was clear and powerful. Her parents started telling her about her birth origins when she was four years old. The young girl referred to her birth as her "special beginnings." They continued to talk about her origins on an ongoing basis, which she said helped normalize it for her. She referred to her surrogate mother as her "carrying mother," and her mother as her "caring mother." The audience asked her many questions.

She delivered a key message to parents who had gone through infertility treatment to have their kids. Her story was about being open and building trust, and included the following components. She told us to start talking with our kids early. She told us to make the story part of the "fabric of the family life." That helped her feel that the surrogate process was not abnormal. It felt okay and normal for her. She felt ongoing love and unquestioned acceptance and support from her family. They put together a scrapbook for her and shared it with her, and she said this was helpful for her as well. She felt secure in herself and who she was. She also told us that she had never had anybody say anything negative to her after learning about her birth history. She had shared this information with some of her friends. I thought to myself, if my daughter turned out to be anything like this young girl, I would be very proud of her.

Finally, there are a couple of other components that can

contribute to making this disclosure bridge more successful. If you do choose to share this information with your child, make sure you have armed him or her with the skills and tools needed to know what to do with this information. Let them know who you have told, so they are not caught off guard. There may be people they want to talk with about it, but they are not certain who knows and who does not. If family members or friends are not immediately told, and find out later, they may also have some negative feelings towards you, the parents, for not telling them.

One possible response suggested by a friend at the seminar was to just say, "We felt it was our child's story to tell, when he or she was ready to tell it." When it is appropriate, you can share with your child the thought process you used around disclosure. Talk to the child about who you told, why, and why not? Let the child decide who else the information will be shared with. Let them know that there is no stigma attached to this information, but that they can chose to keep it private if they want. Sometimes, having control of this information is important to kids, and this can carry forward into adulthood, too. Ultimately, your child should have ownership of their disclosure as an adult, and you should respect their wishes.

The bottom line is: if a child is given the proper skills and tools, and parents choose to disclose the child's genetic origins, it can be a very positive experience for all concerned. The main message to continuously give your child is that they are loved, they are wanted, and that you are incredibly grateful that they are a part of your life. Let them know that you look forward to the days ahead with them. If the proper foundation is laid and continuously built on and developed, your child will ultimately emerge with a strong sense of self-worth and self-esteem. Be as honest as you can with your child, and that will open the door for the child to be honest with you. Remember, you will be modeling this type of behavior as a parent. The rewards can be great for all concerned.

CHAPTER 18
MENOPAUSAL MOMS

Statistics show that women are waiting longer to have children. For people who are struggling with infertility, that wait can be a lot longer than they originally intended. I thought it was worthwhile to take a look at some of the advantages and disadvantages of being an older parent because this sometimes goes hand-in-hand with having infertility treatment.

My husband and I were talking one day. I had begun throwing the covers off in bed because of my hot flashes. This was very uncharacteristic for me because I am one of those people who is always cold. I also noticed I was a bit moodier than I usually am. I tend to be a fairly even-tempered person. He looked at me and said, "So, let me get this straight. I have a wife going through menopause and a daughter who is going through the terrible twos." With a tinge of fear in his eyes, he looked at me and asked, "Just how long does menopause last?" I smiled and said it could be years—many, many years. He just shook his head and had a faraway look in his eyes. Several of the mothers I know are in a similar situation. We are going through menopause, one of the final rites of passage for women, while we are diapering and changing our babies. What impact does all of this have on us as parents?

I thought it would be helpful to get insights about this issue from some of the people I interviewed. I asked them to discuss the pros and cons of being an older parent. I talked with Kate and Eric about it. Kate said: "In some ways it is really great and in some ways it is really hard. I am aware of the fact that I am one of the oldest moms here. Then I look around and say I am only seven or eight years older than these moms. This is mostly in day care situations. I am in a different place than all of them with my job and my career. What is more divisive is that I am not a full-time mom but a full time employee. They are heading off to raise a family...It is hard to go back to your friends who are married and have no children and click with them or my friends who are married and have kids in college. To find families that are similar to yours in age and experience and then have a young one—it is unusual and it is nice when it happens."

Eric added, "I am really sure that I am ready to be a parent. At age twenty I wasn't ready to be a parent. You have your whole life to think about 'what if.'"

Sue and Howard had some additional thoughts. Sue said: "Financial is a big advantage, just in general—having more money to support a child. I don't think we had any level of self awareness like this in our twenties. We were able to impart all of this stuff to our toddler...I was so stupid when I was twenty-five and knew nothing about myself or how to deal with people. He is going to be much better off having these parents. That is so much more important than the down side in that we are going to be so much older as he grows up. When he is graduating from high school, I would much rather be raising an emotionally healthy child, than be able to run around and play football and not know what the hell I was doing. We don't do as much personally. Our social life is less and the energy we have for each other is less. That's hard."

Howard said, "The advantage is more knowledge and more patience for us. We spend a lot of time with him and the energy level is different."

I thought Sue's final thoughts really said it all. At the end of our interview she said: "It doesn't matter if they are biologically yours or not. I say that because I used an egg donor but I also know people who have adopted and had their own. Everyone is a parent in the same way. They love their children the same. I wouldn't close off options in the beginning. Parenting is so incredible in any way you come about it. Prepare to be exhausted from both infertility treatment and parenting."

My husband and I talked a lot about being older parents. Both before we had our daughter and after she was born. My perception was similar to Sue's. I feel we both have a lot more to offer her as older parents. My husband and I both did extensive traveling and also went to college and I did graduate work. I was able to establish myself professionally for many years. He also has been able to pursue his work and continues to do new things professionally. Neither one of us looks back and can name something we wish we would have done that we haven't done.

We bring all of the knowledge, wisdom, and experience we got from our earlier lives to our daughter now. I am certain she will be a richer and better person for it. This would not have been the case if I had a child fifteen or twenty years ago. I don't feel I have anything left to prove to myself professionally at this stage of my life. We are fortunate in that we have some financial security. This is another thing we can offer our daughter now that we might not have been able to offer her if we were a lot younger. I am able to devote myself to spending time with my daughter on a full-time basis. My husband works from home. She most certainly is emotionally and developmentally enriched by having both of her parents be able to spend a lot of time with her.

BALANCING LIFE CHANGES

It can be an interesting and challenging time for you as an older parent as well. Having a child later in life can give you the opportunity to take a time out from your career. You may leave a job or career you were not totally happy with. This time out gives you a chance to be with your child and re-examine the career choices you have made. You may decide to branch out in a different area or try something new in terms of a career. For example, I began doing volunteer work for RESOLVE and started writing again. This can be a surprisingly rewarding realm for some of us that might not have considered making the switch without the addition of a child in our lives.

Obviously not everybody has the option of choosing to stay home on a full-time basis. It is a luxury to be sure. But those of us like Kate, who balance work and parenting, are better equipped to do this juggling act because we are older and more experienced in terms of managing our time and trying to manage our lives.

There is another important component in this equation of weighing the pros and cons of being an older parent. Over the years we have developed a very strong and loving community of friends in addition to our families. This group of people is an integral part of our lives and the life of our daughter. She loves them dearly and views them as family and they also love having her be a part of their lives. These long-term, strong relationships have been built up over the years. They are a cherished part of our world and one of the rewards of getting older. As our lives move in and out of other people's lives, if we are lucky enough, we find good people along the way. They are people who see us through a lot of ups and downs and are there for us no matter what happens. It takes a long time to develop these special friendships. Their presence in our lives nourishes us and makes us better people and ultimately better parents. Their presence also impacts the quality of my daughter's life.

Family involvement can be different for older parents. Our parents are older; many are retired and more settled in their lives. They may have more free time. This may give them the opportunity to spend more time with their grandchildren. Grandparents have unique things to offer our children. This relationship is a reciprocal one. Everybody learns and benefits from time spent together.

It is important to also highlight some of the negative aspects of being an older parent. When children enter your life as an older parent, sometimes you may need to think about uprooting your life. If you have been living in the same place for a long time and you have a child, it may necessitate changes. You may need more space in your home. You might need to move from an area where you have felt comfortable and built a support network. Maybe the neighborhood you live in does not have a good school system, and you will be forced to think about moving to an area that offers a better, more affordable education for your child.

The financial piece can ultimately be a negative as well as a positive. Older parents may have to think about paying for college at a time in their lives when they were planning to retire. In an uncertain economy this can be a big financial burden and a major future stressor.

For many people who have been working for fifteen or twenty years, the transition to being a stay-at-home mom or dad can be difficult. You suddenly find you are not interacting with your peers on a regular basis. There is an element of social isolation, too, because it is harder to spontaneously go out with your friends like you did before. You do not have the ongoing intellectual challenges and stimulation you might have gotten from your job. The way your day is structured is totally different. The physical demands are different. Your internal body clock is broken. You are up at all different hours and often can not adhere to the sleep patterns you had become acclimated to. Parenting can seem more exhausting than work, and without the tangible rewards that come with the end of a day. The parenting day, in fact, never ends, and this can add to the sense of fatigue and purposelessness that people who stop working can feel.

If you are going from a stimulating career to staying home, you will need to allow yourself time to adjust to all of this. You should realize this transition is a significant adjustment, and it is normal to feel a bit disoriented in the early stages of the parenting process. Many people expect that spending time with their baby will be wonderfully fulfilling, and while this is true, staying home with your baby can also be burdensome. Our high expectations for fulfillment can be sorely disappointed.

As we age, changing our routines can become more difficult because our bodies and our minds have established some set patterns of reacting and thinking. Be aware of this and prepare yourself for it. Think about how you react to change. Think about how to keep doing some of the other things that have been important in your life. Explore new ways you can approach your emerging role as a parent, and remember you have more flexibility to incorporate a variety of pursuits into your day-to-day life. Many older parents come to appreciate the freedom being home provides them. For people who have worked their entire adult life, this freedom can seem to lack structure and be disorienting, but it can also be a rare opportunity to create your own pattern of occupations. You can pursue a rich variety of rewarding endeavors that can serve both you and your child. You both need external stimulation, and you will both thrive on daily routines that provide for this.

MORTALITY AND OLDER PARENTS

One of the critical issues that older couples often struggle with is the fear that, as an older parent, there is a greater likelihood that one of them could become ill or die suddenly. Younger parents rarely worry about cancer or heart disease, but older parents often have peers they know who are struck suddenly. The older we get, the more we witness mortality among our peers. Like many older parents, my husband and I struggle with this issue and the burden it could place on our child. We are particularly aware of it, because we have only one child. My husband and I have talked about the special challenge that may place on our daughter in the future. Clearly, as older parents, we are farther along in our life expectancy, and there is a chance we will not be there in the future to share in all our daughter's major life events. As we age, we could also become a burden to her.

Obviously none of us have a crystal ball, and we don't know what the future holds. I don't believe it helps to dwell on this type of thinking. But I do think it is imperative to give it some serious thought. First, it is important to make the proper legal and caretaker provisions for your child, so that, in the event anything happens to you and your partner, it is clear who will take care of your child. You should consider how your child will be provided for should you die or become seriously ill or disabled. Conversely, you should consider how you can provide for your own needs, when your child becomes an adult. It is tremendously important to try to alleviate as many of these potential future burdens as we can for our children.

As older parents, illness or disability can arise for us at a time in our child's adult life when he or she is just trying to forge a career or build some type of personal or financial independence. A lack of preparation can create great personal conflicts for your child or children, if the burden of your lack of planning falls to them to address. The possibility of your earlier mortality is also an issue with the potential to have a tremendous impact your kids' lives. Losing a parent is particularly trying, no matter your age, but the younger you are, the harder it can be. When it is appropriate, you do need to share your wishes and values regarding your own mortality. This is an all-important issue to address with your child. Your children need to be old enough to understand the difficult and complex issues associated with living their lives after their parents are gone.

When your child is old enough, it is best to have this conversation before anything happens. You need to be able to have an open and frank dialogue with your child, preferably while this conversation is still "safe" to have. Let your child know what type of safeguards you have in place. There should be other adults they can turn to in a crisis to get help, guidance, and support. You should make as many decisions in advance as you can and document these in writing, including medical directives and your funeral desires. You should also try to provide financially for these needs in advance. Don't leave the burden of these decisions to your kids, and let them know about your wishes face to face. Your kids need to know how to make the decisions that may need to be made, and they should be supported in this process. There should be a place where you have this all down in writing. Your child needs to know where to find this and how to access it. Nobody likes to think about death, serious illness, or crisis, but you do want to have some sort of viable plan in place for the sake of your child. It is a special gift to give.

KEEPING UP WITH KIDS

There is no denying that as we get older, our energy level is not the same as when we were younger. Women's hormone levels are changing, which can contribute to fatigue. One of the biggest challenges about being an older parent can be just physically keeping up with your child. I heard about a research study shortly after my daughter was born and never forgot it. They took several athletes who were marathon runners and in excellent shape, and had them spend the day with a bunch of two-year-olds in a day care setting. Their task was simple. They were assigned to imitate all of the movements of a particular two-year-old. The athletes were to mirror everything the kids were doing, and they tried. The athletes collapsed after two or three hours. They just couldn't keep up.

This is not surprising for those of us who have kids that age. It made me feel a little better knowing that—no matter what kind of shape I was in—it was natural for me to have times when I was exhausted. That combined with a lack of sleep can be just the thing to make us feel like we are dragging ourselves around. I have found that the best thing I can do is try to pace myself and my daughter. I try to provide opportunities for my daughter to run around and play every day as much as possible so that it will help her get tired and ultimately nap. Her napping gives me a chance for some down time as well which is useful for both of us.

Nap time can be a critical part of recovery for mothers, particularly when our babies haven't established night-long sleeping patterns yet. Many mothers build up sleep deficits, because they follow their normal adult patterns for going to sleep, but then get up during the night or earlier than normal in the morning because of their kids. In general, small children need more sleep than adults, but they tend to get a lot of sleep while their parents are awake. By taking naps or going to bed earlier, they get a head start on their parents. Many parents share the burden of sleep deprivation and "take turns" at night, but more often than not, it is mothers that build up the most significant sleep deficits.

Supervising small children can require a lot of vigilance, and it is often difficult to get anything else done. Many moms view nap time or the early bedtime of their children as the time of the day to "get things done." Instead of stopping, maybe taking a nap themselves, they try to do as many things as they can while their kids are asleep. Sometimes moms stay up later for the same reasons. This can be an issue for all moms, but it is especially critical for older women. Good sleep patterns get more important to our health as we age. Sleep deprivation is a major source of stress. You should be aware of your sleep needs, and realize that, if you've lost sleep, it's a good idea to try to catch up again by napping when your child naps, or turning in early. As I pointed out earlier, menopause can also disrupt sleep. It's not easy being an older parent with small children, but one of the critical ways to "keep up" with them is keep up on sleep.

There is something else women can do for themselves. This advice is found in *Family Building* magazine and comes from an article by a therapist named Nancy London. Ms. London specializes in women's health issues, and she has some special insights to offer women who become parents after the age of forty. She tells us: "Women in their forties need downtime, time to rest and to reflect on what's coming up in the second half of their lives. These are legitimate needs, but it's hard to justify filling them when we've waited so long to be a parent. It seems selfish. It's important for women to put themselves on the list of the people they nurture. One way they can do this is through the support and encouragement of other women who are also trying to find a healthy balance in their lives... It's one of the reasons support groups are so important."(36)

She goes on to highlight one of the hardest things about being an older mother: accepting our age. She writes: "The most difficult thing to do is to admit what you are feeling and own it. The problem with that is that we live in a youth-worshipping culture. People are telling us we have to get nipped and tucked to be acceptable as a mom. There are no models out there telling us to accept our bodies and accept the changes."(37) Pregnancy does change us physically. We gain weight and often our bodies change shape. The experience can seem to accelerate the aging process, and getting back to "the shape we were in" before pregnancy can be extremely challenging, if not impossible. For many women, this never happens. But that doesn't mean we are necessarily any less healthy or attractive. We are different; we are older—there's no denying it. Being happy and accepting of ourselves as we are is a big component of our attractiveness, particularly as we get older.

My belief, after spending time with many women who are older mothers, is that they are not afraid of their age. They are willing to take risks and make personal sacrifices for things they really believe are important. These women do not let age stop them from doing something that they really want to do, like making it possible for a child to become a part of their lives. These older women are not afraid to do things that may be against societal norms. The fact that they are willing to become a mother at this later stage in their life lends credence to that statement. They have the necessary self-confidence to be different, to do what they do, and be who they are! The menopausal mom is to be celebrated!

I also agree with Ms. London, however, that we women are notoriously bad at taking care of ourselves. We put other people's needs in front of our own. She is right that we need to remind ourselves that our needs are legitimate as well. By helping to nurture ourselves and keep ourselves strong and healthy, this will ultimately help us to feel better about ourselves and bring more quality into the lives of the people around us. And that especially includes our partners and children!

C H A P T E R   1 9
BECOMING A COUPLE AGAIN

One of three things will happen as a result of your undergoing infertility treatment. You will learn you are not able to have a child. You will have a child through collaborative reproduction, IVF techniques, or adoption. You will decide to remain childfree. No matter which of these outcomes is yours, you and your partner will be going through it together, and your relationship will be perhaps one of the few constants in your infertility journey. Obviously, whatever happens, it will have an impact on your relationship. There may be times when your bond feels stronger, and times when it feels stressed and quite fragile, depending on how you cope with infertility as individuals and as a couple. Whatever the circumstances of your outcomes, you and your partner will likely need to spend some time learning how to be a couple again. Infertility is a lot to go through, and whatever your outcome, there will be a time of adjustment and reorganization associated with it.

In earlier chapters we talked about how the infertility journey can become an obsession. As Eliza put it, the pursuit can "have an addictive quality to it." The quest to have a child becomes all-consuming, and we are often willing to put all else aside to make it work in any way we possibly can. When you think about it, even before we have a baby on the way, we are already totally focused on that baby and building our lives around it. We are making personal, physical, emotional, relationship, and career sacrifices to make our quest for a child work.

The journey itself changes us as individuals and as couples. There are times of crisis that test us. You may deal with a crisis in an entirely different way than your partner. Sometimes, we can each seem to be alone in the struggle, out of synch, or at odds. We discussed this in the chapter on the psychology of infertility. There may also be times of incredible happiness and joy that you and your partner will share. These heightened moments will belong to both of you and bind you more strongly together. Sometimes, hard times can provide the same intensified belonging through shared empathy and sorrow. Whatever happens, you will be tested individually and jointly along the way. Making decisions will test your communication skills, your values, and your knowledge of yourself and your partner.

Let's look at how couples are challenged and respond to the outcomes that leave us childless. If you ultimately learn you cannot have a child or if you choose to be childfree, what will be the implications for you and your partner? You will have both put a lot of time, money, physical, emotional, and psychological energy into trying to have a child. You will have sacrificed a great deal, hoping a child would become a part of your lives. Letting go of this dream will involve a grief process, as we discussed in Chapters 10 and 11. You may grieve in different ways and adjust to the loss of your imagined child in different ways. The picture you had of your future world included a family for you, your partner and child (or children). Now you and your partner recognize that the family will be the two of you. There may be feelings of blame, sadness, disappointment, anger, or shame. These feelings may relate to the cause of your infertility, and they can turn a functional relationship into a dysfunctional one.

You will need to be open to working through these feelings individually and together as a couple. To make this work, there has to be some form of viable communication between the two of you. If you can't find ways to talk about it effectively with each other, think about seeing a therapist who can help give you the skills and tools you need to move beyond this point. Again, if you do decide to see a therapist, I would recommend seeing somebody who specializes in working with people who have infertility problems.

Healing often requires you to have a shift in your focus. You will need to construct a future orientation that recognizes your immediate family will be just you and your partner. There will be a lot of introspection involved, as you put aside some of your earlier dreams about building a family. Your life post infertility treatment can be a rich and fulfilling life. Your task is to think about the ways to make it as wonderful and productive a life as you can. One way to look at what has happened is that your life has taken a different path than you originally intended it to take. Think about the things in your life that brought you the most joy before you started your infertility journey.

Think about your courtship with your partner. What were the things you did that helped bring you closer together? What things did you and your partner do that made you a strong team when you were engaging in your battle against infertility? Is it possible to do those things now? What qualities in your partner were the most helpful to you as you went down the infertility path? How can those qualities bring a new depth and richness to the current and future relationship between the two of you?

Your childfree lives will have some significant changes. You will have more day-to-day freedom and the flexibility to travel. Your physical health may be better now that you don't have to use medications that might have caused physical or emotional discomfort or instability during your treatment. Your sexual relationship can have a new spontaneity and freedom that was not possible while you were under the infertility treatment microscope. You can try to create new ways to recapture your intimacy. Perhaps, once you have made the decision to be childfree, you will ultimately feel less stressed.

Allow yourselves more time to nurture yourselves as individuals and as a couple. You may have felt the need to isolate yourselves while you were in the midst of your infertility treatment. When you feel ready, begin to break down some of these barriers you may have created to protect yourselves. Be sure to include time for you to be alone together on regular basis. Sometimes this requires designating an agreed upon time for quality togetherness. Also, allow time to be with friends or family, and seek out the people you feel most relaxed and comfortable with. For a time, this may mean other people without kids, or you may be comfortable around children, too. Consider what situations will feel most comfortable for you individually and as a couple. Be sure to talk about this with your partner before you make plans with others. It's okay to go slowly at first, but over time you should try to get back to the wider social circle of regular life.

You may have more financial freedom now than you had anticipated you would, and this can offer you new opportunities. Perhaps, there is a class you had hoped to take some day that you now have the time and the money to pursue. There might be things you can do together or things you want to do for yourself. Your relationship will now be exclusively as husband and wife, without the additional role of parent. Spend some time thinking about what your relationship as a couple means to you, and look for ways you can help strengthen it, so it can grow and endure. It may ultimately become stronger and closer than you might have imagined.

THE PARENTING COUPLE

For people who have kids through infertility treatment or adoption, there are also a lot of adjustments that must be made. The addition of a child or children into your family changes the whole dynamic of your family. Your marital relationship now does not necessarily feel like it is the number one priority anymore. In fact, it is rarely the number one priority at all. That is a shock to many people. We spend so much time thinking about having a child that, when it finally happens and the child comes into our lives, we are not certain about what to do. Our priorities change and they seem to take on a momentum of their own, as though there is little choice left.

Our young children do need our constant attention, and they often require our ongoing focus. They do become the center of our lives. They rely on us for everything and we do what we can to meet their needs. While we are learning to adjust and take care of our kids, we are doing it with ongoing sleep deprivation. We are also in this state of utter awe and amazement that this thing that we have dreamed about and hoped for would happen—has happened—and we can't believe it. How does all this impact our relationship with our partner?

One major change that occurs is that, while on the infertility journey, you and your partner are working as a team towards a common goal. You are usually in agreement about how to get there. This can change after a child arrives. There will be a whole host of new decisions to make, and life can seem to remain unsettled for long periods of time. You may engage in power struggles about how much attention the child should get and from whom. You may have different opinions about child rearing techniques. Where should the baby sleep? How often should the baby eat? How often should the baby be held? Who should, and how do you, get the baby to stop crying? Whose job is it to change the diapers? How will the other chores at home be done and by whom? With multiple decisions to be made on a near-daily basis, there is lots of room for disagreement as you figure out how to tackle these new challenges. Communication can suffer when people are sleep deprived, and, in conjunction with this, they can become more short-tempered. Conflicts can impact intimacy, as can fatigue, and without quality intimacy as a couple, disagreements can easily begin to cycle into ongoing conflict.

When we imagine what type of parents we will be, it is often based on our own personal experiences with our parents and their parenting styles. If asked, you could probably talk about what things your parents did that you liked, and what things they did that you vowed you would never do if you had children. Are you or your partner doing some of those things now? Have you and your partner talked about your families and how you envision parenting well together? Is your idea about your parenting style the same as your partner's idea? Are you or your partner particularly sensitive to certain parental behaviors, and have you discussed how to be aware of these and avoid them? Are the differences in your parenting styles great enough to cause conflict between you? How is that spilling over into your marital relationship?

The moment that children enter your life, it feels like your time is no longer your own. The time demands from your children are great. Sometimes you need to sleep when your child does, just to try to recharge yourself. You may feel torn in many directions trying to be a caretaker to your child, take care of the chores and responsibilities at home, and perhaps at work. Juggling all of this is tough and can be a source of great stress and pressure. How much time does that leave for you to give to your relationship with your partner?

Take some time to think about and look at how becoming a parent affected your relationship as a couple. Did it bring you closer or farther apart? Did it make you more independent or more dependent on your partner? Did it give you more or less financial independence? Did it affect your work or career in a negative way or positive way? Has it improved your communication or made it worse? Why? How did all of these things impact your relationship with your partner? Were these expected or unexpected outcomes? Were you aware of these changes before now? How did you react to them?

Becoming parents can disrupt many aspects of life. Some people become convinced that everything has to change at once. Now that they have a child, they need to move to a bigger house or a nicer neighborhood. The cost of living goes up as parents, sometimes dramatically. The change over to a family lifestyle can have big, ongoing financial impacts, particularly if one partner stops working and your combined incomes falls. Couples often find they have more costs and less money. Financial constraints can force them to do things they don't want to do or can seem to limit the choices. When one partner has been working and stops, they can suddenly feel dependent on the other partner for the first time. This can make a host of decisions more difficult and generate conflict. Money is one of the most important sources of conflict in couples, and sometimes issues around money don't surface until there's a shortfall relative to perceived needs. When people become parents, their perceived needs change, and sometimes their income stream, too. It's good to keep these variables in mind, as you look at how to maintain a healthy relationship as a couple.

As you face the many challenges of becoming parents, there are some things that you can do to get your relationship with your partner back to where you want it to be. Communication is the first thing, and sometimes this requires setting aside a time to sit down and talk. Sometimes it helps to make this a more formal process, something that happens regularly, on schedule. Some people continue this as a family practice as their kids grow up. You want to be sure that each person participates by bringing up issues and sharing in their resolution. This shouldn't just become a forum for complaints, and if it ever degenerates into blaming a "timeout" should be called. The focus should be problem-solving and making mutual decisions. Good listening is important, as is an ongoing willingness to compromise. Having kids requires more shared decisions, and you can develop skills for this as a couple.

Another thing you can do is to allow both partners to take an active role in the parenting activities with your child or children. If your partner works during the day maybe, he or she can be the one to give your child a bath or a shower at night. Bath time is one of my husband's favorite times with our daughter. She loves it, too, and they relish this time together. Sometimes it is hard as a mother to relinquish some of the tasks we do regularly. It is important to positively reinforce your partner's willingness to participate in your child's care. Maybe a sock will go on inside-out when your child is getting dressed. You need to let go of some of those things. It will give your partner a great deal of satisfaction to share in some aspects of the care giving role with your child. It will help strengthen your partner's bond with your child. Another end result of sharing this role is that it will strengthen your bond with your partner. You may also find that one of you is better at a task than the other, and it will be a relief to share some of these responsibilities. It will also give you and your partner something to talk about and share together.

As you embark on your new role as a parent, it will feel like your world does revolve around your child. And, indeed, a lot of your time and energy should be focused on your children. But you still need to make room in this world for the two of you as a couple. It is imperative to make some time—and take some time—for the two of you to be alone and focus on your relationship together, apart from being parents. This is no easy task. You both will be feeling tired, with periods of very low energy, and it won't always be easy to make that extra time. But making it can bring a much-needed boost to your relationship with your partner. This time should not be spent talking about your child and what he or she did today. It should be used instead to nourish your relationship as a couple.

Talk to each other about how and what you are doing as individuals. Try to do some things to re-establish intimacy that may have been lost in the previous months. Have an agreed upon time to have fun together, once a week or every other week, and set this aside just for the two of you. If you can afford it, get a babysitter and have a date night, where you treat yourselves and get out of the house. If one partner stays at home most of the time, going out can be particularly beneficial. If going out is not a possibility, set some time aside when your child is asleep to do something special together. Maybe a family member or neighbor can watch your child, while you go for a long walk. You can have a nice meal, a quiet bath, some good music, a massage. Figure out what feels right for the two of you, and allow yourselves this time to make it happen. It will bring a dimension to your relationship that many people unexpectedly lose after they have children.

For couples who have a child after infertility treatment it is so easy (and tempting) to get totally wrapped in your child's world. You have yearned for so long to have this opportunity, and you want to relish every moment of it. But remember, strengthening your relationship as a couple will ultimately strengthen your parental relationship with your children. The love, respect, and affection you show for each other as a couple serves as a wonderful model for your children. It is something that will stay with your child throughout his or her life. They watch you carefully and observe the way you relate to each other. You will see this as your child gets older and begins to do imagination play. You will see it in the way your child interacts with his or her toys and dolls. Watch how your child touches the toys, talks to the toys, disciplines the toys, and interacts with the toys. Our children hold a mirror up to us, and we can see our reflections in it. What would you like your child to see in that mirror? What would you and your partner like to see in that mirror? Those are important questions to consider.

Whatever the outcome of your infertility experience, much of your future quality of life will depend on your relationship with your partner. Being in a supportive relationship improves health and increases happiness. All couples face challenges over time, and will need to adapt to stay together. The roller coaster ride of infertility can be particularly hard on relationships, and this remains as true afterward, whatever your outcome. Whether you are childless or become a parent, a new life journey begins. Sometimes this involves letting go of dreams, and at other times it involves adapting to the reality of the way dreams come true. Either way, it's usually not what we expect. Adjusting expectations, changing dreams, reorienting life—these are all challenging to the dynamics of a couple. Healthy couples work together to adapt. They find ways to communicate, resolve conflicts, support each other, and maintain intimacy. Sometimes, this takes real work, but however challenging it is to start a new life journey together, it can also be the source of future growth and renewal and happiness.

CHAPTER 20
SOME FINAL THOUGHTS ON THE RIDE

This summer I took my daughter to an amusement park. We went with a friend who also has a daughter as a result of infertility treatment. We ended up taking a ride on one of those chute roller coasters that ends up splashing in water. Kids my daughter's age and size were allowed to ride it. I hate roller coasters and haven't ridden one in over twenty years. We slowly inched our way up and I thought this isn't so bad. Suddenly we were at the top of a forty foot drop. Our car began falling down the tracks. My heart raced, my anxiety level shot up, and my head throbbed. I had my daughter in a death grip. We made it to the bottom of the ride and hit with a big splash, before gently floating into the stopping point.

My friend and I staggered out of the chute car. We were shaken. Our girls jumped up and screamed, "Let's do it again and again." I thought: *let's try another ride* (not a roller coaster). There was a giant pirate ship that moved back and forth like a pendulum. We climbed on that, and as it began to rock back and forth, I lost my stomach on the second swing. I closed my eyes praying it would end soon, and hoping that keeping my eyes shut would ease my suffering. It didn't! My friend and I got off that ride and I looked at her and said, "The things we do for our kids. I'm sure that's not the last time we'll do something for them we would never do otherwise." She nodded and smiled knowingly. It was also somehow comforting to have my friend there with me going through it. She totally understood what I was thinking and feeling without me saying much of anything.

I thought about that day as I began to write this last chapter. There is the obvious parallel of the roller coaster, which I use as a metaphor throughout this book. I thought those rides that day really did mirror infertility treatment for me and many others. I would do something that terrified me, that wreaked havoc on my body and my mind for my child. I would take what I perceived as a personal risk for her. When I knew I couldn't handle the roller coaster anymore I chose another ride, hoping that different ride would work, and it would please her and end successfully for both of us.

Those of you reading this book will be in many stages along your infertility journey. There will be days when things will go well, when test results are promising, or when you actually learn that you are pregnant. The day may finally come when it is time to leave and go bring home your newly adopted child and start your family. You may get word from your clinic that they have found a donor match for you or that a surrogate has been identified who will help make your dream of becoming a parent come true.

There will also be days where your test results will show that you are not pregnant. And days when you learn the medication you have been taking is not working, and you will have to try something new. Perhaps, you will continue to be unsuccessful at getting pregnant, and your physician won't be able to identify the reason for your infertility. Maybe you will get to the point where you feel that if you have to undergo one more needle prick you will scream. You may ask yourself what is wrong with you or your partner—or what "bad thing" you did—that you are unable to create a child, no matter how many treatment options you use.

There may also come a day when you and your partner decide to stop infertility treatment and begin your post-treatment life, choosing to live childfree. It may be hard to imagine this day coming, depending on who you are, and where you are in your infertility journey. Not everyone succeeds, but life can have many fruitful outcomes.

All of these scenarios are emotionally charged. Whatever happens to you and your partner as you continue along the path of your infertility treatment, you can be certain you will be forever changed by your infertility experiences. Your relationships with your partner, your family, and your friends will also be impacted by your infertility experience. Your infertility will challenge and perhaps change these boundaries. You will be forced to make difficult decisions along that way that will test you in new ways. Your infertility journey may cause you to question your own instinct and your judgment. It will force you and your partner to look deeply inside yourselves to understand and define your values, religious beliefs, and life choices. By definition, the need to undergo infertility treatment creates a life crisis.

My hope for you is that you also recognize that you do not

need to be a passive passenger on this difficult infertility journey. After reading this book, I hope you can and will be able to assume an active role. If you have a doctor that does not seem to be meeting your needs, you can find another one. You can hire an attorney to offer you information and provide you with the legal protection you need as you negotiate surrogate, adoption, or donor arrangements. Remember, you do not need to go through infertility treatment alone. If you are having difficulty coping with the challenges that arise, you can seek counseling on an individual or support group level. There are lots of places to go to get the specific information that you need to make informed decisions along the way. Friends and family can be educated by you and your partner, and if you enable them, they can help you meet your needs as you proceed through your infertility journey.

The surprising part about the challenges of infertility is that facing them can become an empowering experience for you. You will need to arm yourself with the proper tools, knowledge, and support systems. Don't be afraid to rely on existing support systems or, if necessary, you can help build new support systems to aid you and others to get to where you are going. Allow yourself the flexibility you need to alter your course along the way, as your circumstances change. Your infertility journey may help you achieve a new and greater level of intimacy with your partner, your family, and certain friends. Your ability to overcome the crisis that may occur can strengthen you. You may make new and lifelong friends along the way. You can actively determine if and when your journey comes to an end. Give yourself permission to look at and consider all of the options that are available to you. Take comfort in knowing that the number of treatment options available to you is growing. The technology, science, and research are ongoing, and ever changing. As doctors gain a greater understanding of the realm of infertility, the success rates for infertility treatment are improving. There is no reason to think that this trend won't continue.

There is no doubt that, wherever and whenever you emerge from your infertility journey, you will be forever changed. There is no way to know the outcome or what it will make of you. You will certainly be changed in ways that you had not considered when you began. The person you become as a result of this experience will be better equipped to deal with other life challenges that will undoubted-ly arise in the future. The resiliency of the human spirit, and the poten-tial capacity that we all have to cope with uncertainty and crisis, is something that has never ceased to amaze me in my many years of work as a social worker.

My hope and wish for you is that, wherever your own person-al infertility journey ultimately takes you, it is a place you can accept and look forward from. Whatever our outcomes, we all need to find a future direction where we want and choose to go. My wish is that, wherever this leads for you, it ultimately offers you some sense of peace, belonging, and fulfillment.

C H A P T E R   2 1
GLOSSARY OF TERMS RELATING TO INFERTILITY

I don't know about you, but I know that for me the complex terminology of infertility was confusing. When I entered the world of infertility treatment, the doctors and nurses and support staff that I worked with were speaking a language that I didn't always understand. This surprised me, because I did have a long history of working in the healthcare profession. One thing I learned about infertility treatment is that this is so cutting-edge that new treatments and medications are being developed all of the time. This constant innovation brings new medical terminology, incomprehensible abbreviations, and a host of new and confusing words. You will likely be mystified and feel that real understanding is incredibly complicated to break down.

Don't let all this overwhelm you. This language is second nature to your reproductive endocrinologist and the staff at you infertility treatment center or clinic. When you hear or see a word you don't understand, stop the person you are working with and ask that person to explain it. Don't let them off the hook until they explain it in a way that you are sure you understand. If you are reading something that doesn't make sense, bring it to a doctor or nurse, and ask them to serve as your interpreter. There is nothing wrong with admitting you don't understand something. The other part of this is that you will be given certain information that is packaged in a way that feels foreign to you, and then you will be asked to make incredibly difficult decisions. In order for you to make the right decision, you will need to understand this base of information, and how it specifically applies to you. So, it is vital that you understand the facts that are put before you in order to move on to the next step.

I have included this glossary as a guide to help you along the way. It is by no means complete or definitive. As I write this, new medications and treatments are being used and this list will already be out of date. The technology is changing too quickly. But I though it would be helpful to have a short glossary to use as a guide through this maze of infertility language. I have tried to focus on terms I have seen in articles, heard through my treatment, and used in my book. There are examples that came up in discussions with friends who were having infertility treatment. I have also tried to take the most common terms, and explain them briefly and simply. If you hear a term from your healthcare practitioners that is not on this list, be sure to ask for clarification, and write down their explanation. These things can be quickly forgotten, and sometimes it helps to keep your own, personal glossary. I hope this glossary can serve as a useful starting point for you.

GLOSSARY OF TERMINOLOGY RELATING TO INFERTILITY

Abdominal ultrasound aspiration: A procedure done to remove an egg from the ovary. An aspirating needle is pushed through the abdominal wall into the ovarian follicle to retrieve the egg.

Acrosome membrane: A cover over the head of the sperm which has specific enzymes that, when they are released, allow the sperm to penetrate the egg.

Acrosome reaction: A breakdown of the membrane above that causes the sperm to change into a cell that can penetrate into the egg.

Adhesions: These are bands of scar tissue that attach the surfaces of different organs to each other. They can be found in connection with fallopian tubes attaching to the ovary.

Aggultination: When a bunch of sperm bond together.

Anovulation: An inability to ovulate.

Antisperm antibody test: A test that can determine if antibodies on the sperm are impeding the mobility of the sperm, the ability of the sperm to fertilize the egg, or their ability to penetrate through the cervical mucus.

Asherman's syndrome: When scar tissue forms in the cavity of the uterus and inhibits normal uterine lining development.

Assisted hatching: An opening made in the embryo to facilitate the implantation or attaching of the embryo to the lining of the uterus.

Assisted Reproductive Technologies (ART): A term used to describe infertility treatment procedures such as IVF and GIFT.

Asthenospermia: A word used to identify the condition of sperm having limited mobility.

Azoospermia: A medical condition where is no sperm present in a man's semen.

Basal Body Temperature (BBT) chart: A daily record of the temperature of your body when it is in a restful state. It is a way to determine when you are ovulating, because your body temperature rises slightly at the time of ovulation.

Blastocyst: When the sperm and the egg have come together, forming an embryo that has cells that will make a placenta and cells that will become a fetus. It takes five to six days to create a blastocyst.

Capacitation: This occurs after ejaculation, when the sperm travels through the reproductive system of a woman, and causes the sperm to be unable to penetrate the egg.

Cervix: A small opening connecting the uterus to the vagina that produces mucus, which lets sperm pass into the uterus.

Chorionic villus sampling: A sample of cells taken from the placenta, usually done at the beginning of your pregnancy.

Chromosome: A structure in every cell's nucleus that contains the genetic information or the DNA (deoxyribonucleic acid) of the parent.

Clomid: A fertility medication given to women to stimulate ovulation. It can be used with men to help the production of sperm.

Collaborative reproduction: When a couple decides to use donor gametes (eggs or sperm) from another person as a means of getting pregnant. In terms of surrogacy, when a surrogate agrees to carry and give birth to a child.

COH: Excessive stimulation of the ovaries.

Computer assisted semen analysis (CASA): When computers are used to measure the amount of sperm, the shape of sperm, and how they move.

Donor insemination (DI): The sperm from a donor is put in the woman's uterus or cervix during ovulation.

Dyspareunia: Discomfort or pain while having intercourse.

Ectopic pregnancy: When an embryo implants outside the uterus.

Egg aspiration: The removal of an egg from a follicle on the ovaries during an in vitro fertilization process.

Egg donation: The aspiration of the eggs from a donor, who volunteers to help another woman get pregnant.

Embryo: This is the term used for a fertilized egg until it reaches the eighth week of pregnancy.

Endometrioma: A condition where infection causes inflammation in the ovary.

Endometriosis: A condition when the uterine lining becomes infected and inflamed.

Endomitrium: The tissue that lines the inside of the uterus.

Estradiol: Estrogen that is formed and released by ovarian follicles at the time of ovulation.

Extracorporeal fertilization: Another term for in vitro fertilization. This is fertilization of the egg that is done outside of the woman's reproductive tract.

Fallopian tubes: Two tube-like structures that connect to the uterus. These tubes carry the eggs from the ovary to the uterus. The tubes are where the egg and sperm get together and begin the fertilization process. After fertilization, the egg moves from the fallopian tubes into the uterus.

Fecundity rate: A woman's ability to become pregnant during any month when ovulation occurs.

Fertilization: The moment when the egg is entered by the sperm.

Fibroids: Non-cancerous tumors made up of fibrous tissues that can be found in the uterus.

Follicles: Sacks of fluid that can be found on the ovary, which help eggs get ready for release at the time of ovulation. They are also a source of estrogen production in women.

Follicle-stimulating Hormone (FSH): A hormone made and released in the pituitary gland. FSH is the source of the stimulation of follicle growth in women and sperm production in men.

Gamete: An egg or sperm reproductive cell.

Gamete Intrafallopian Transfer (GIFT): An assisted reproductive technique where eggs and sperm are removed, placed together, and put into the fallopian tubes.

Gestational surrogate: A woman who agrees to carry an embryo/fetus that has no genetic relationship to her, in order to assist another woman who is not capable of carrying a child through a pregnancy.

Gonadotropins: Medications that are injected. Their purpose is to help begin ovulation. They have a combination of follicle stimulating hormones and luteinizing hormones. Examples are Pergonal and Gonal F.

Gonadotropin-releasing hormone: A hormone that controls the production and release of FSH and LH.

Hormone Replacement Therapy (HRT): Some women use HRT after menopause to combat serious problems with hot flashes, night sweats, and shedding of the uterine lining.

Human Chorionic Gonadotropin (HCG): A hormone made in the placenta during pregnancy. It is used during ovulation-induction therapy to help promote the release of the egg.

Human Menopausal Gonadotropin (HMG): A medication used during fertility treatment that consists of LH and FSH.

Hydrosalpinx: A part of the fallopian tube swells and fills up with fluid.

Hysterosalpingogram (HSG): A high level x-ray study that is used to take a picture of the fallopian tubes to determine if they are damaged in any way. It also can take a picture to see if the uterus appears all right.

Hysteroscopy: A small, thin telescope that is placed in through the cervix and used to see into the uterus to determine if there are any problems.

Implantation: When the embryo is attached to the lining of the uterus.

Infertility: The inability to get pregnant after trying for a year with unprotected intercourse.

Intracytoplasmic Sperm Injection (ICSI): This is done in the laboratory when eggs and sperm are retrieved from the woman and the man. One sperm cell is placed in the egg and then this fertilized egg is transferred into the woman's uterus.

Intrauterine Insemination (IUI): A technique where sperm is placed directly into the cervix or the uterine cavity.

In vitro fertilization (IVF): An assisted reproductive technique where eggs are removed from the ovary and sperm is also taken from the man. The two are then combined for fertilization in a laboratory. After the fertilization is completed, the resulting embryo is placed into the uterus.

Karyotyping: A blood test for assessing the chromosomes of a man and a woman.

Laparoscopy: A procedure where a small, narrow, telescope-like instrument is inserted through the abdominal wall or belly button.

Lupron: A medication used to suppress hormone levels.

Luteal phase: This begins when the woman starts to ovulate and can be detected by higher levels of estrogen and progesterone.

Luteinizing Hormone (LH): A protein found in the pituitary gland which is used in the process of ovulation.

Male factor infertility: This is when the cause of infertility is due to problems with the man's sperm and/or when these problems combine with a woman's infertility problems create an inability to conceive a child.

Micromanipulation: A highly technological procedure where an instrument is used to help in vitro fertilization.

Microsurgical Epididymal Sperm Aspiration (MESA): A surgery designed to collect large amounts of sperm.

Oligospermia: This is a sperm count so low an egg cannot be fertilized.

Oocyte Maturation Inhibitor(OMI): A protein in the fluid of follicles that stops the egg from maturing.

Ovarian failure: This is a problem with the ovaries, where there are no follicles or eggs, or they do not respond to FSH stimulation.

Ovarian stimulation: When fertility medications are used to increase the number of eggs produced, and it can also help regulate single egg ovulation.

Ovaries: The female reproductive organs where eggs and sexual hormones are made.

Ovulation: When the egg is released from the follicle.

Ovum: A female egg.

Pelvic Inflammatory Disease (PID): An inflammation of the uterus, ovaries, and fallopian tubes which can result in infertility in women at times.

Pergonal: This is a mixture of FSH and LH used to enhance follicle activity.

Polycystic Ovarian Syndrome (PCOS): A medical problem where multiple cysts found in the ovary can cause a hormonal imbalance, which in turn causes potential problems with menstruation and ovulation.

Postcoital Test (PCT): A test that is done soon after intercourse to find out if there is a problem with the sperm's ability to move through mucus found in the cervix area.

Preimplantation genetic diagnosis: This involves removing a cell from the embryo before it is placed in the uterus to examine and to determine if there are any genetic abnormalities.

Premature ovarian failure: When a woman's ovaries stop producing estrogen and she is then unable to ovulate. This is caused by early menopause.

Progesterone: A hormone that is made after ovulation begins. It is a key hormone that helps maintain pregnancy at the beginning.

Retrieval: The retrieval of eggs by use of a probe inserted through the vagina and moved to the ovary. Follicular fluid is removed and place in a syringe. Eggs are identified by lab staff and placed in a culture medium where they will be combined with sperm.

Round Spermatid Nucleus Injection (ROSNI): A relatively new experimental technique where cells are removed from the testicles and then the genetic material in the nucleus is placed into an egg.

Salpingitis Isthmica Nodosa (SIN): A disease that causes a blockage in the fallopian tubes. It sometimes can be repaired by a surgical procedure.

Sonogram: This is a test where high-frequency sound waves are used to show pictures of structures inside the body.

Sperm: The man's reproductive cell which is produced in the testes and released into the semen.

Spermatocyte: An underdeveloped sperm cell.

Subzonal Sperm Insemination (SUSI): A procedure where a tiny device is used to inject sperm into the egg.

Testosterone: The predominant male hormone also found in women.

Tubal Embryo Transfer (TET): A technique where an embryo is put into the fallopian tube after in vitro fertilization.

Urofollitropin (FSH): This is FSH that is used to enhance follicle growth and maintain development.

Uterus: The major female reproductive organ used to protect and maintain the fetus.

Varicocele: A dilated vein in the scrotum that can contribute to reduced quality of sperm and also impact the quantity of sperm produced.

Zift: An egg is retrieved via ultra-sound aspiration, following this procedure a newly fertilized egg is returned to the fallopian tube.

Zygote: An egg that has been fertilized.

Zygote intrafollopian transfer: When a fertilized egg is put into a fallopian tube.

CHAPTER 22
INFERTILITY RESOURCE INFORMATION

In this final chapter I wanted to spend some time giving you information on places that you can go to find information that may be useful to you in your infertility journey. We are lucky in that there are a growing number of resources out there. When I began my research for this book I was very surprised at the wealth of information available.

I did want to say something about the Internet. Many people use the Internet as their source for most of their information. When I went on the Internet to do some research for my book I saw literally thousands of sites. I just want to caution you about these web sites. Some of them can be incredibly useful and full of helpful, up-to-date information. Other web sites can be put together by people you don't know and the information they contain may not be totally accurate or credible. There are chat rooms available, which can be a great source of support for people. There you can chat with other people who have had similar experiences with infertility problems and treatment. Keep in mind that what works for them might not work for you.

If you get information from the Internet try to check it out with a healthcare professional or trusted friend or family member who may have knowledge about it. People create web pages for a multitude of reasons. We know that you can now go on-line to look for an egg donor or sperm donor. People are placing advertisements for all kinds of things on the Internet. You can find information about infertility clinics around the country and adoption programs around the world. Again be cautious until you have information about the people you are dealing with. You want to make sure that their motives are honest and that they have the ability to help you achieve your goals in a safe and appropriate way.

Please remember that some of the organizations I list may have local chapters near you. Check your local information sources or go on-line if you can to find out addresses that may be closer to your area. Your local infertility clinic, hospitals, RESOLVE, adoption agencies, doctors, nurses, or therapists specializing in infertility may also be a good source of information for you.

RESOURCES

NATIONAL AND REGIONAL ORGANIZATIONS

Adoptive Families of America
3333 Highway 100 North
Minneapolis, Minnesota 55422
612-537-0316

American Academy of Adoption Attorneys
P.O. Box 33053
Washington, DC 20033

American College of Obstetricians and Gynecologists
409 12th Street SW
Washington, DC 20024
202-638-5577

American Fertility Society
1209 Montgomery Highway
Birmingham, Alabama 35216
205-978-5000

American Society for Reproductive Medicine
1209 Montgomery Highway
Birmingham, Alabama 35216
205-978-5000
email: asrm@asrm.com

The American Surrogacy Center
638 Church Street NE
Marietta, Georgia   30063
770-426-1107

Center for Loss in Multiple Birth, Inc. (CLIMB)
P.O. Box 104
Palmer, Arkansas 99645

Compassionate Friends
P.O. Box 1347
Oak Brook, Illinois 60521

Endometriosis Association
8585 North 76ᵗʰ Place
Milwaukee, Wisconsin   53223
1-800-992-3636

Ferre Institute
258 Genesee Street Ste 302
Utica, New York 13502
315-724-4348

International Council on Infertility Information Dissemination
(INCID)
P.O. Box 91363
Tucson, Arizona 85721
520-544-9548

National Adoption Center
1218 Chestnut Street
Philadelphia, Pennsylvania   19107
1-800-TOADOPT if you do not live in Pennsylvania
In Pennsylvania call 215-925-0200

National Adoption Information Clearinghouse
1400 Eye Street NW, Suite 600
Washington, DC 20005
202-842-1919

National Committee for Adoption
1930 17ᵗʰ Street NW
Washington, DC 20009
202-328-1200

National Council for Adoption
1930 17ᵗʰ Street NW
Washington, DC 20009
202-328-1200

Only Child Association
9810 Magnolia Ave.
Riverside, California 92503
909-689-6865

RESOLVE, Inc.
1310 Broadway
Somerville, MA 02144
617-623-0744
www.resolve.org

Society for Assisted Reproductive Technology (SART)
1209 Montgomery Highway
Birmingham, Alabama 35216
205-978-5000
email: asrm@asrm.com

The American Infertility Association
666 Fifth Avenue Ste 278
New York, New York 10103
888-917-3777
www.americaninfertility.org

The Childfree Network
7777 Sunrise Boulevard #1800
Citrus Heights, California 95610
916-773-7178

The Organization of Parents through Surrogacy (OPTS)
7054 Quito Ct.
Camarillo, California 93012
805-482-1566

The Society for Reproductive Endocrinologists (SRE)
1209 Montgomery Highway
Birmingham, Alabama   35216
205-978-5000
email: asrm@asrm.com

The Society for Reproductive Surgeons (SRS)
1209 Montgomery Highway
Birmingham, Alabama 35216
205-978-5000
email: asrm@asrm.com

PERIODICALS

Family Building
RESOLVE
1310 Broadway
Somerville, Massachusetts 02144
www.resolve.org
email: resolveinc@aol.com

Fertility Weekly
1087 Crooked Creek Road SE
Eatonton, Georgia 31024
www.holonet.net
email: kkey@hendersonnet.atl.ga.us

INCIID Insights
International Council on Infertility Information Dissemination
P.O. Box 91363
Tuscon, Arizona 85752
520-544-9548
www.inciid.org
email: INCIIDinfo@aol.com

Newsletter of RESOLVE National
1310 Broadway
Somerville, Massachusetts 02144
617-623-0744
www.resolve.org
email: resolveinc@aol.com

Only Child News
137 N. Larchmont Boulevard
Los Angelas, California 90004
www.onlychild.com
email: onlychild@earthlink.net

BIBLIOGRAPHY

This bibliography also serves as a listing for footnotes. Sources are listed by chapter, and alphabetically by author.

CHAPTER 1: What is Infertility?

Clapp, Diane N., R.N., B.S.N., "Guidelines for Making the Change to an Infertility Specialist," *Family Building* ,Volume 11, Issue #2, Winter 2003, RESOLVE p. 25.

Deveraux, Laura, Hammerman, Ann Jackoway, *Infertility and Identity: New Strategies for Treatment,* San Francisco, California: Jossey-Bass, 1998, pp. 78, 79.

Johnston, Patricia Irwin, *Taking Charge of Infertility* ,Indianapolis, Indiana, Perspectives Press, 1994, pp. 19, 25.

Manning, Barbara Eck, *Guide for the Childless Couple,* New York, New York, Prentice Hall Press, Simon & Schuster Inc., 1988, p.101.

Marrs, Richard, M.D., Friedman-Bloch, Lisa, Silverman, Kathy Kirtland, *The Fertility Book,*
New York, New York, Delacorte Press, 1998, p. 417.

CHAPTER 2: Finding Your Doctor

Marrs, Richard, M. D., Friedman-Bloch, Lisa, Silverman, Kathy Kirtland, *The Fertility Book,* New York, New York, Delacorte Press, 1998, pp. 65, 69.

Ory, Steven J., M.D.," Moving from an OB/GYN to a Reproductive Endocrinologist,"*Family Building*, Volume 11, Issue #2, Winter 2003, RESOLVE, p. 9.

CHAPTER 5: Health Insurance and Paying for Treatment

Marrs, Richard, M.D., Friedman-Bloch, Lisa Silverman, Kathy Kirtland, *The Fertility Book*, New York, New York, Delacorte Press, 1998., p. 362.

Michaelsen, Barbara Frank, Wachenheim, Deborah, "*Questions to Ask When Choosing an Insurance Policy #35*," National RESOLVE Handout, 1998.

CHAPTER 6: Legal Issues

Clapp, Diane N., R.N., B.S.N., "Questions to ask When Signing Consent Forms or Contracts", *Family Building*, Volume 11, Issue#3, Spring 2003, p. 27.

Jain, Tarun, M.D., Harlow, Bernard L., PhD, Hornstein, Mark D., *New England Journal Of Medicine*, Volume 347, August 29, 2002, pp. 661-666, "In The News,"*Hope*, RESOLVE of Illinois, Volume 24 #5, Holiday Issue 2002, p. 17.

CHAPTER 7: Making the Decision to Stop Treatment

Johnston, Patricia Irwin, *Taking Charge of Infertility*, Indianapolis, Indiana, Perspectives Press, 1994, pp. 152, 154-155.

Kluger-Bell, Kim, MFT, "Mourning the Losses of Infertility," *Family Building*, Volume 1, Issue #4, Summer 2002, RESOLVE, pp. 10-11.

CHAPTER 9: Adoption Considerations

Hughes, Michelle, M.,JD, "Adopting Across Racial Lines," *Hope,* RESOLVE of Illinois, Volume 24, #2, Spring 2002, p. 18.

Johnston, Patricia Irwin, *Taking Charge of Infertility,* Indianapolis, Indiana, Perspectives Press, 1994, p. 196.

McDermott, Mark T., JD. "Legal Aspects of Adoption," *Family Building,* Volume 11, Issue #3, Spring 2003, p.20 ,21.

CHAPTER 10: Making the Choice to Live Childfree

Kluger-Bell, Kim, MFT, "Mourning the Losses of Infertility," *Family Building,* Volume 1, Issue #4, Summer 2002, RESOLVE, pp. 10-11.

CHAPTER 11: The Psychology of Infertility

Deveraux, Laura, Hammerman, Ann Jackoway, *Infertility and Identity: New Strategies for Treatment,* San Francisco, California, Jossey-Bass, 1998, pp. 202-203.

Mahlstedt, Patricia P., Ed. D., "The Psychological Component of Infertility," *Fertility and Sterility,* Volume 43, #3, March 1985, p.336-337, p. 345.

Manning, Barbara Eck, *Guide for the Childless Couple,* New York, New York, Prentice Hall Press, Simon & Schuster, Inc., 1988, pp. 111, 115.

Marrs, Richard, M.D., Friedman-Bloch, Lisa, Silverman, Kathy Kirtland, *The Fertility Book,* New York, New York, Delacorte Press, 1998, p. 383.

CHAPTER 12: Building a Support Network

Johnston, Patricia Irwin, *Taking Charge of Infertility,* Indianapolis, Indiana, Perspectives Press, 1994, pp. 48-50.

Mintle, Linda S., Ph.D., "When Families Let you Down," RESOLVE of Virginia, April 1996, p. 7.

CHAPTER 14: Parenting after Infertility

Johnston, Patricia Irwin, *Taking Charge of Infertility,* Indianapolis, Indiana, Perspectives Press, 1994, pp. 223, 225, 226.

CHAPTER 17: Disclosure

Baran, Annette, Pannor, Reuben, *Lethal Secrets: The Shocking Consequences and Unsolved Problems of Artificial Insemination,* New York, New York, Warner Books, 1989.

Bernstein, Anne C., *Flight of the Stork: What Children Think and When about Sex and Family Building,* Indianapolis, Indiana, Perspectives Press, 1994.

CHAPTER 18: Menopausal Moms

London, Nancy, "Coming Late to Motherhood," *Family Building,* Volume 1, Issue#3, Spring 2002, RESOLVE, p. 21.

INDEX

Wyatt-MacKenzie is excited about this new magazine that shares our mission of supporting moms.

total 180!

THE magazine for the professional stay-at-home mom.

Check it out at: www.total180mag.com

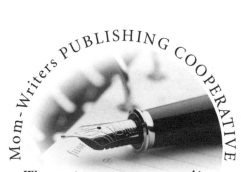

We empower mom writers.

Publishing the Works of Extraordinary Mom Writers

Wyatt-MacKenzie Publishing, Inc.

WyMacPublishing.com